Contents

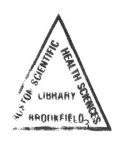

Acute Care 2004

A national survey of adult psychiatric wards in England

In association with the National Institute for Mental Health in England Acute Inpatient Care Programme

Ines Garcia
Claire Kennett
Mansur Quraishi
Graham Durcan

ISBN: 1 870480 63 5

Published by

The Sainsbury Centre for Mental Health
134-138 Borough High Street
London SE1 1LB

Tel: 020 7827 8300
Fax: 020 7403 9482
www.scmh.org.uk

The Sainsbury Centre for Mental Health (SCMH) is a charity that works to improve the quality of life for people with severe mental health problems. It carries out research, development and training work to influence policy and practice in health and social care. SCMH was founded in 1985 by the Gatsby Charitable Foundation, one of the Sainsbury Family Charitable Trusts, from which it receives core funding. SCMH is affiliated to the Institute of Psychiatry at King's College, London.

A charitable company limited by guarantee registered in England and Wales no. 4373019

Charity registration no. 1091156

Design by Intertype

Printing by Nuffield Press, UK

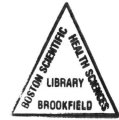

118638880

118638880

Foreword

Malcolm Rae and Paul Rooney, Joint National Programme Leads

National Institute for Mental Health in England (NIMHE)

Acute Inpatient Care Programme

The response to this survey has been encouraging, which firmly indicates a widespread desire to seek improvements. There are many positive messages emerging, which demonstrate the commitment and resourcefulness of those involved in acute care. The report also highlights some serious concerns, which frustrate those endeavouring to provide an effective service to people who are often vulnerable and have complex needs.

The way the information is presented will assist regional comparison with national figures. We hope the findings will stimulate national, regional and local debates, enable an evaluation of priorities and resources, and prompt an assessment of current standards and practice to trigger further local audit and service improvements.

We are delighted with this initiative, as we believe the information provided really does add value to the challenge of raising the profile of the acute speciality to achieve a better experience for those who use or work in acute care services. We anticipate that the report will act as a spur to service development and complement the many other initiatives currently underway.

We expect the document will promote a dialogue between service providers, users and commissioners, which can lead to a closer understanding of the main concerns and dilemmas and assist in developing a unified, structured and coherent strategy for developing acute services.

The reader will find many gems in the report and we point to one notable area concerned with the workforce. At first glance, there is an array of recommendations sufficient to frighten those at present engaged in what might be perceived as an avalanche of imperatives and pressures. However, under closer examination the report focuses on current established topics of concern and developments, and if followed through in the way envisaged, will be helpful in signposting and supporting a way through the potentially overwhelming challenges. We suggest that this information should feature in local Agenda for Change discussions.

We suggest that giving proper attention to these issues, by emphasising the need to work together with other interested parties on the issues of local concern, will ensure benefits.

Now is the time to tackle many of these issues, to address the need for a well-led, motivated, self-confident workforce and refresh the drive for service improvement. The challenge is to find ways to use the findings of this report in a creative way and be associated with a service that is progressing forward.

Acknowledgements

This report would not have been possible without considerable input from a number of people from a range of organisations. Where job titles are shown, it should be noted that these relate to the time of involvement with the project. The authors would like to thank:

Ward managers, Trust chief executives and other staff

First and foremost we thank 310 ward managers nationwide for taking the time to complete the ward survey and we also thank the many trust chief executives and their colleagues who provided information for the staffing survey.

For assisting in the questionnaire design: Trust-based staff

Central and North West London Mental Health Trust

Sylvia Barry, Acute Inpatient Care Project Manager
Gus Malahleka, Katie Allatt, Mac Manzini, Suna Smythe, Eugine Yafele and Lisa Lowe, Project Site Leads

South Downs Health NHS Trust

Ian McLuckie, Ward Manager, Regency Ward, Mill View Hospital

Camden and Islington Mental Health and Social Care Trust

Adam Dorman, Ward Manager, Mornington Unit (PICU), Huntley Centre, St Pancras Hospital

The Hillingdon Primary Care NHS Trust

Ken Hikwa, Ward Manager, Adult Mental Health Unit (Riverside Centre)
John Adadiaha, Ward Manager, Adult Mental Health Unit (Riverside Centre)
Zita Sibre, Ward Manager, Adult Mental Health Unit (Riverside Centre)

For assisting in questionnaire reviews/pilots: Staff at the following Trusts

Isle of Wight Healthcare NHS Trust
North West Surrey Mental Health Partnership NHS Trust
East London and The City Mental Health NHS Trust
Coventry Teaching PCT
Newcastle, North Tyneside and Northumberland Mental Health NHS Trust
Selby and York PCT
West Sussex Health and Social Care NHS Trust

For expert advice, comment and reviews:

The Sainsbury Centre for Mental Health (SCMH)

Steve Clarke, Programme Lead for Acute Care
Dr Jed Boardman, Senior Policy Advisor

Dr Frank Keating, Senior Research Fellow, Breaking the Circles of Fear
Lesley Warner, Senior Researcher
Malcolm Philip, Director of Workforce Development
Tony Powell, Senior Researcher
Tina Braithwaite, Project Manager, Acute Solutions
Tabitha Lewis, Programme Lead in Dual Diagnosis
Andy Bell, Director of Communications
Julie Hadman, Publications Manager

Royal College of Psychiatrists' Research Unit

Maureen McGeorge, Audit Manager

Health Advisory Service (now Health and Social Care Advisory Service)

Geoff Brennan, HAS consultant and City Nurse Researcher, City University, London

National Institute for Mental Health in England (NIMHE)

Malcolm Rae, Joint National Programme Lead, NIMHE Acute Inpatient Care Programme
Paul Rooney, Joint National Programme Lead, NIMHE Acute Inpatient Care Programme
Yvonne Stoddart, National Programme Manager, NIMHE Acute Inpatient Care Programme and Acute Lead North East, Yorkshire & Humber Development Centre
Dr Richard Ford, Director, South East Development Centre
Mary Munday, Acute Programme Lead, South East Development Centre
Gemma Hughes, Programme Director, London Development Centre
Paul De Ponte, Senior Public Health Information Analyst, London Development Centre
Dr Hugh Middleton, Acute Care Lead, Associate Director, East Midlands Development Centre and Senior Lecturer, University of Nottingham, Division of Psychiatry
Bill Peacham, Acute Care Programme Manager, East Midlands Development Centre
Nick Adams, Acute Programme Lead, West Midlands Development Centre
Phil Minshull, Acute Programme Co-ordinator, North West Development Centre
Alan Howard, Development Consultant in Acute Inpatient Care, South West Development Centre
Denise Hall, Associate Consultant in Acute Inpatient Care, South West Development Centre
Robert Humphreys, Associate Consultant in Acute Inpatient Care, South West Development Centre
Lou Brewster, Service Improvement Lead, Eastern Development Centre
Tom Dodd, Primary Care and Community Teams National Programme Lead
Colin Gel, Service User Department Lead, East Midlands Development Centre

Project Steering group

Dr Tony Ryan, Service Development Manager and Senior Research Fellow, Health and Social Care Advisory Service (and author of *A Survey of NW Acute Ward Managers*)

Donna Fraher, Project Service User Advisor

Graham Saxton, Project Service User Advisor

Nick Adams, Acute Programme Lead, West Midlands Development Centre, NIMHE

Colum Clinton

Mike Gill, Development Officer, Modernisation Team, Hull & East Riding Community Health NHS Trust

Yvonne Stoddart, National Programme Manager, NIMHE Acute Inpatient Care Programme

Malcolm Rae, Joint National Programme Lead, NIMHE Acute Inpatient Care Programme

Paul Rooney, Joint National Programme Lead, NIMHE Acute Inpatient Care Programme

Claire Kennett, Joint Project Manager and Project Analysis Lead, SCMH

Ines Garcia, Joint Project Manager and Project Research Lead, SCMH

Mansur Quraishi, Information Analyst, SCMH

Graham Durcan, Senior Consultant Analytical Services, SCMH

For allowing the reproduction and use of data:

Mental Health Service Mapping for Working Age Adults (Durham University)

Professor Gyles Glover, Director of the Centre for Public Mental Health, University of Durham

For the provision of London acute ward details:

Len Bowers, Professor of Psychiatric Nursing, City University, London

About NIMHE and the RDCs

The National Institute for Mental Health in England (NIMHE) was launched in 2002 and aims to improve the quality of life for people of all ages who experience mental distress. It helps all those involved in mental health to implement positive change, providing a gateway to learning and development, offering new opportunities to share experiences and one place to find information.

NIMHE is made up of eight Regional Development Centres (RDCs), whose role is to support staff and local stakeholders to put policy into practice and to resolve local challenges in developing mental health.

The Acute Inpatient Care Programme is one of NIMHE's core programmes aimed at generating local action, promoting and sustaining service collaboration and continuous improvement in the delivery of acute inpatient care and in its connections and integration with other key elements of the wider system of health and social care.

Each RDC has an acute care lead appointed to work with provider trusts, commissioners, local implementation teams (LITs), service user, carer and voluntary organisations, those responsible for local and national monitoring, education and training organisations, and other relevant bodies, to deliver the programme aims.

Many of the figures in this report show results at RDC level and we have abbreviated the names of the RDCs as follows:

National Institute for Mental Health in England (NIMHE)	
Regional Development Centres	**Abbreviations used**
Eastern	East
East Midlands	EMids
London	Ldn
North West *	NW
North East, Yorkshire and Humber	NY&H
South East	SE
South West	SW
West Midlands	WMids

*It should be noted that the North West region did not take part in the ward survey (see methodology for further details).

Introduction

The *Mental Health Policy Implementation Guide: Adult Acute Inpatient Care Provision* (DH, 2002a) describes acute inpatient care as a

> "core and integral component of the *National Service Framework for Mental Health* to which all the NSF standards are relevant. Improving adult acute inpatient care and its connections and integration with the other key elements of the whole system of care in its local context is a priority NSF implementation target."

It is crucial that we understand and acknowledge this essential role of acute inpatient care if mental health services are to provide high quality seamless care to those who need it. This survey attempts to offer a snapshot of acute inpatient services in 2004: a 'benchmark' by which future improvements stemming from the *National Service Framework for Mental Health* (NSF-MH) and the subsequent policy implementation guidance can be measured (DH, 1999a). It provides that snapshot through a survey of ward managers and mental health trust chief executives across England.

Considerable investment has gone into developing community mental health services and alternatives to hospital admission, the NSF-MH being only the most recent driver in the move from the old Victorian asylums to the community-focused services of the present day. The number of mental health beds has greatly reduced since the 1950s and may be expected to fall further in coming years with the introduction of new types of community team such as those which help people in a crisis.

The impact of these developments is already being felt in many acute wards. Early evidence, cited later in this report, on the impact of these new teams, suggests that the inpatient population profile is changing. Ward staff report working with people who have a greater severity of mental health problems than they previously experienced. This is a predictable consequence of providing intensive home-based mental health care to prevent admission wherever possible. It means that, more than ever, the acute inpatient ward is a place offering critical assistance to people during episodes of extreme psychological distress and impaired functioning.

If they are to fulfil their respective remits successfully, acute inpatient wards and community teams must work together. This interdependence is a critical factor when services are implementing any new initiatives, such as social inclusion or race equality, or when new guidance is created. Without understanding and valuing the role of acute inpatient care in these initiatives, services risk only ever partially achieving their aims for a service user-focused and equitable service.

Within this whole system, each part has its own challenges and we cannot gloss over those facing acute inpatient care. Recruitment and retention of staff is just one area of difficulty which can be exacerbated by a lack of career opportunities in acute inpatient care, insufficient training designed for acute inpatient staff, high staff sickness and high bed occupancy. All of these problems create a pressured and demoralised workforce (SCMH, 1998; Higgins *et al.,* 1999; DH, 2002a; Glasby & Lester, 2003; Clarke, 2004). On top of this, neglected or inappropriate acute inpatient buildings and a lack of adequate facilities can exacerbate the problems in trying to provide a comfortable and therapeutic environment (The Royal College of Psychiatrists, 1998a; SCMH, 1998; DH, 2002a). Published in 2004, Mind's *Ward Watch* survey of current and recent inpatients (including acute wards) highlighted a number of key concerns for service users on wards including safety, the therapeutic environment, staffing and accommodation (Mind, 2004).

In drawing attention to the challenges and difficulties that confront those providing acute inpatient care we should not forget that there are already initiatives, both national and local, underway to build upon or improve the quality of services. As a result of the guidance for adult acute inpatient care we have seen the setting up of acute care forums (ACFs) and these play an important part in developing and implementing service improvement plans. Positive practice in acute inpatient care needs to be shared. In addition to work carried out by ACFs and other networks, the virtual Knowledge Community created by NIMHE is one way this is being taken forward. Much work is being done to tackle complex issues such as the recent publication of guidelines on *Violence: The short-term management of disturbed/ violent behaviour in in-patient psychiatric settings and emergency departments* (NICE, 2005).

The *Acute Care 2004* survey has been a collaboration between The National Institute for Mental Health in England (NIMHE) and the Sainsbury Centre for Mental Health (SCMH). The exercise has been an ambitious one, surveying every acute inpatient ward individually and senior management in every mental health provider trust in England. In carrying out the survey, we have worked closely with the Regional Development Centres (RDCs) of NIMHE, experts in the field, users of mental health services, acute care forums and ward managers and staff.

The survey had two questionnaires, one that was sent to acute inpatient ward managers and one that was sent to trust chief executives. Ward managers have a key and central role in acute inpatient care and are in a position to provide data on a wide range of subjects. Just over two thirds of all acute inpatient ward managers in England completed the survey, giving us a wealth of information on issues such as ward environment, cultural sensitivity, the impact of community teams, the operation of the Care Programme Approach (CPA), staff training, and the therapeutic and leisure activities provided to service users, to name but a few. The second, shorter questionnaire, for chief executives, related to ward staffing, bed occupancy and staff sickness and we received a similar response to this from trusts in England.

These high response rates indicate a real willingness from health service staff to be involved in shedding light on the current state of acute inpatient care. This enables both the positive and negative aspects of acute inpatient care to be seen and moreover provides an essential baseline from which to measure the impact of subsequent changes. We have also been able to present the findings in the report by region, through which RDCs can identify particular issues in their regions and with which individual trusts can compare their own services.

No survey can provide a complete picture of inpatient care and the *Acute Care 2004* report forms part of a wider programme of work for both NIMHE and SCMH, which is aiming to do just that. There are a number of high profile programmes of work already underway such as 'The Search for Acute Solutions', a project being undertaken by SCMH to address the issues highlighted in the *Acute Problems* report (SCMH, 1998). City University is conducting the 'City-128 Study of Observation and Outcomes on Acute Psychiatric Wards' that is designed to investigate the use of special observation and other containment measures employed by nursing staff on acute psychiatric wards. The National Patient Safety Agency (NPSA) is running the 'Patient safety programme to safeguard mental health service users', and the Royal College of Psychiatrists' Research Unit is conducting 'The National Audit of Violence: towards safer and more therapeutic residential care for people with mental health problems or learning disability'. These are just some of the projects and there are, of course, a number of smaller but equally valuable regional and local initiatives being undertaken around the country.

The importance of this *Acute Care 2004* report is that it gives, for the first time, a national baseline from which we can gain an overview of the key areas for further work. It should provide useful reference points (benchmarks) for those commissioning and providing mental health services, and indeed other stakeholders. These benchmarks can be revisited to monitor the ongoing implementation of the NSF-MH and other initiatives. The report should also prompt action to address the gaps and concerns identified and be used to inform service improvement priorities.

Abbreviations	
ACF	Acute Care Forum
AOT	Assertive Outreach Team
BME	Black and Minority Ethnic
CBT	Cognitive Behavioural Therapy
CHI	Commission for Health Improvement (as of 31 March 2004 all functions taken over by the Healthcare Commission)
CMHT	Community Mental Health Team
CMHSD	Centre for Mental Health Services Development (now HASCAS)
CPA	Care Programme Approach
CPAA	Care Programme Approach Association
CRT	Crisis Resolution Team
DAT	Drug Action Team
DH	The Department of Health
FCE	Finished Consultant Episode
HAS	Health Advisory Service (now HASCAS)
HASCAS	Health and Social Care Advisory Service (merger between the Health Advisory Service [HAS] and the Centre for Mental Health Services Development [CMHSD])
HC	Healthcare Commission
HCA	Health Care Assistant
HES	Hospital Episode Statistics
HR	Human Resources
LIT	Local Implementation Team
MH	Mental Health
MHA	Mental Health Act
MH-PIG Adult Acute	The Mental Health Policy Implementation Guide: Adult Acute Inpatient Care Provision
NHS	National Health Service
NICE	National Institute for Clinical Excellence
NIMHE	National Institute for Mental Health in England
NPSA	National Patient Safety Agency
NSF	National Service Framework
NSF-Children	National Service Framework for Children
NSF-MH	National Service Framework for Mental Health
OT	Occupational Therapist
PCT	Primary Care Trust
PEAT	Patient Environment Action Team
PICU	Psychiatric Intensive Care Unit
PDP	Personal Development Plan
RCPsych	The Royal College of Psychiatrists
RDC	Regional Development Centre
RMO	Responsible Medical Officer
SCMH	The Sainsbury Centre for Mental Health
SHA	Strategic Health Authority
WDC	Workforce Development Confederation
WTE	Whole Time Equivalent

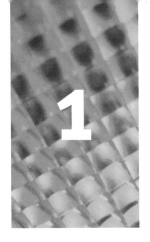

Aims, methodology and limitations

AIMS

The *Mental Health Policy Implementation Guide: Adult Acute Inpatient Care Provision* acknowledges that a service mapping exercise is required to clarify staff and service user profiles for the wards and to identify baseline benchmarks (DH, 2002a). The aim of the *Acute Care 2004* project is to provide this information and create reference points from which ongoing benchmarking can take place. From our findings, we are able to highlight areas of good practice and where further work or more in-depth investigation may need to be undertaken. At the end of each chapter we have also made a number of themed recommendations. These recommendations are not intended to be definitive nor prescriptive but we hope they may provide and stimulate ideas on what could be taken forward as appropriate.

Findings are presented regionally as well as nationally to assist commissioners, regional development centres (RDCs), acute care forums (ACFs), trusts, ward managers and others to use the information in this report to develop action plans which are helpful in influencing resource allocations, as well using it as a baseline for monitoring change.

To fulfil our aim we needed to ensure the collection of up-to-date and complete data from as many acute inpatient wards as possible and to do this, we sent ward surveys directly to ward managers. There is always a degree of subjectivity in this type of self-reporting but the great value of this information is that it comes straight from those most involved in the day-to-day running of the ward.

METHODOLOGY

This report is based on three main sources of information:

1) A national survey of adult acute psychiatric inpatient wards sent to each ward manager in England in 2004 (ward survey)

2) A national survey of funded establishment and actual staffing levels of adult acute inpatient wards along with some trust-wide contextual data sent to each trust chief executive in 2004 (staffing survey)

3) Hospital Episode Statistics (HES) data for 2002/3.

This data was also supplemented by information sourced from the Adult Mental Health Service Mapping website (http://www.dur.ac.uk/service.mapping/) and the Department of Health performance monitoring website (http://www.performance.doh.gov.uk/performanceratings/2002/specs.html).

Ward survey

The survey asked 146 questions about the ward. It did not have a 'census' day but was completed by ward managers across the country over the time period of late January to early April 2004. It covers a broad range of topics ranging from the information provided to service users on admission through to staff training. All of the Regional Development Centres (RDCs) agreed to wards in their regions taking part in the survey with the exception of the North West. At the request of the acute care leads for the region, the North West was not included in the ward survey as another ward survey for the region had recently been carried out by Dr Tony Ryan on behalf of the Centre for Mental Health Service Development, England (CMHSD). We have, where appropriate, matched the data reported in *A survey of NW Acute Ward Managers: Supporting Acute Care Forums' service development agenda* (NW Acute Ward survey) with that of our national survey and commented upon it in this report (Ryan, 2003). Surveys were sent to ward managers by post with the exception of the East Midlands region where they were individually taken by the acute care lead to wards for completion. Ward managers were asked to provide details on bed numbers and 191 wards provided this. The Adult Mental Health Service Mapping data was used to find missing bed numbers by ward where possible. In total we were able to find bed numbers for 277 wards. Our bed numbers are therefore based on a combination of ward survey data and Adult Mental Health Service Mapping data.

Staffing survey

In connection with acute inpatient care only, this survey asked about funded and actual establishments and vacancy rates for all professions as well as bed occupancy, sickness rates and the details of people of working age in the trust catchment (adult population of the trust). Data was collected for all regions including the North West. These surveys were sent to the trust chief executive for dissemination to the appropriate departments. The most complete data we received was on nursing (including both qualified nurses and health care assistants) and occupational therapy (including occupational therapists [OTs] and OT assistants) establishments and we have only reported on these. It was not possible in many instances for a trust to state the level of input from other professionals on the ward. We also had a very limited response to our question asking about the adult population that the trust served, so we have not reported on this.

Hospital Episode Statistics (HES) Data

HES data is an annual set of data based on the statutory Commissioning Data Set (CDS) that is submitted on a monthly basis by all provider trusts (see http://www.dh.gov.uk/PublicationsAndStatistics/Statistics/HospitalEpisodeStatistics/fs/en for definitions). It was agreed that we would use the most recent year's data available at the time of collection (2002/3) to carry out regional analyses, including the North West, on factors such as length of stay, ethnicity etc. The data for 2003/4 was not available at the time that this report was produced. As the HES data we used refers back to 2002/3, it pre-dates changes such as the development of many of the current crisis resolution teams and early intervention teams etc., and thus provides a good benchmarking baseline for monitoring the impact of new community teams. There are some issues around the completeness and quality of some of the data: for example, the Department of Health states that "data quality is a continuing problem for ethnic data collection with the NHS" (http://www.dh.gov.uk/PublicationsAndStatistics/Statistics/StatisticalCollection/fs/en). However it remains the core means of collecting inpatient activity data across all trusts, and is used for planning purposes by the Statistics Division of the Department of Health.

Development of database and survey tools

With the support of Professor Gyles Glover at the Centre for Public Mental Health, University of Durham, we used the service mapping data to create a database of trusts and adult acute psychiatric wards. Ward and trust information was validated by a variety of sources, the most important of which was the acute care leads in each RDC. In total, 85 mental health provider trusts and 492 adult acute psychiatric wards (excluding the North West) were identified.

The questionnaires used for the NW Acute Ward survey (Ryan, 2003) and the Health and Social Care Advisory Service 2003 report *Improving the Quality of Psychiatric Inpatient Care in London* (London HAS survey), informed the development of our survey tools. Initial drafts of our survey tools were presented to the project steering group, acute care forums, ward managers and acute care leads. The draft survey tools were also posted on the SCMH website with a discussion board to invite feedback. A final draft version was then reviewed/piloted in each of the participating RDCs.

Response rates

Ward surveys and staffing surveys were posted out in January 2004. After an intensive follow-up to this, a final deadline was set in early April 2004 for data collection. The response rate for the ward survey was 68% and for the staff survey was 62%. Variations in the response rates for RDCs are detailed in Table 1. The lower response rate for London was expected as this region had recently taken part in the London HAS survey. The 100% response rate for East Midlands is the result of the individual ward visits by the RDC acute care programme manager. It should be noted that for all regions response rates to individual questions may vary.

Table 1   A breakdown of response rates by RDC for the ward survey

RDC	No. wards sent to	No. wards responding	% response rate
East Midlands	34	34	100%
Eastern	40	23	58%
London	122	56	46%
North East, Yorkshire & Humber	91	71	78%
South East	75	54	72%
South West	53	30	57%
West Midlands	63	42	67%

Completed staffing questionnaires were received from 62% trusts. The data accounted for 303 (or 63%) of acute wards identified nationally.

Table 2   A breakdown of response rates by RDC for the staffing survey

RDC	No. trusts sent to	No. trusts responding	% response rate	No. wards where data available	% wards where data available
East Midlands	5	2	40%	13	38%
Eastern	8	4	50%	27	68%
London	10	8	80%	76	62%
North East, Yorkshire & Humber	15	12	80%	59	65%
North West	9	4	44%	30	42%
South East	15	11	73%	48	64%
South West	8	3	38%	18	34%
West Midlands	15	9	60%	32	51%

Data analysis   For the purpose of this report the steering group agreed that data be reported on at national and RDC level. For the most part, data is presented in percentages. RDCs will be given a complete set of data for their regions. Staffing data has been aggregated, where possible, as a per bed ratio or as a percentage. Calculations per head or per 100,000 population would have been more informative particularly if deprivation figures (e.g. measures such as the income, employment, housing etc. in an area) were also incorporated. However, the main obstacle to such comparisons was the fact that staffing data was not complete for any of the RDCs. Analysis and comparison of data for trusts with complete datasets was beyond the scope of the project.

The steering group, experts within the field of acute care from NIMHE such as acute care leads, service user leads and experts from within SCMH and elsewhere, were asked to review and comment upon the preliminary results from the data analysis. The feedback received has assisted in the production of this report.

LIMITATIONS

We achieved a good overall response rate for the combined surveys of 65%. As our sample is not complete, findings should be taken as indicative rather than conclusive. There are therefore gaps in information both in terms of staffing and ward information and these vary by region. As a result, we have been unable to carry out calculations such as 'per head of population' or introduce calculations relating to demographics such as socio-economic factors. Even so, such calculations would have been best suited to answer questions of equity of services, which is clearly beyond the remit and purpose of this project. However, there is the potential for commissioners, RDCs, strategic health authorities and trusts to do further work in this area.

Whilst service users have provided valuable feedback in their reviews of the report, there is much more work that could be carried out at a local level, such as service user and carer surveys, to supplement the report findings. In many ways, these findings are just the stepping-stones to a greater understanding of acute inpatient care.

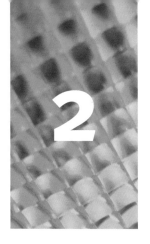

2 Service user and ward demographics

KEY FINDINGS

❖ Our survey showed a national average bed occupancy of 100%

❖ HES data showed the median (midpoint of the range) length of stay varied across the regions from 38 days to 44 days

❖ HES data showed that 34% of service users were coded under the category of 'psychoses' and 49% under the category of 'non-psychoses'

❖ HES data showed that the ethnicity of service users was not always recorded

❖ Our survey showed that 79% of service users detained under the Mental Health Act 1983 were detained under Section 3

❖ 39% of ward managers reported that high intensity/one-to-one observations occurred frequently on their ward

❖ Our survey showed that there was a national average of 3 hours 57 minutes of escorted leave per ward on the day that the ward managers completed the survey (day of completion varied)

❖ 4% of beds in our survey were used solely for detoxification

---

CONTEXT

This first chapter aims to give a broad understanding of service user and ward populations. Information for this section comes from three sources: the ward survey (details about the ward were requested directly from ward managers); the staffing survey (details of staffing numbers and bed occupancy were obtained from trusts via their chief executives); and Hospital Episode Statistics (HES). Where our findings state at the 'time of the survey' this relates to the period when the ward managers filled in their survey during late January to early April 2004.

Hospital Episode Statistics (HES) Data

Information about service users such as their ethnicity, diagnosis etc. is coded and entered into trust information systems. This information is submitted to the Department of Health and published as Hospital Episode Statistics. We have used the latest available statistics at the time of the report production and these relate to the year 2002/3. It is to some extent inevitable that there will be coding errors in such a large amount of data and we did find some coding errors during our analysis such as the use of incorrect ethnicity code, inaccurate lengths of stay and diagnoses. These are discussed in each section of this chapter as appropriate.

WHAT WE FOUND

Bed occupancy

In 1998, the Royal College of Psychiatrists published a working party report that states "to operate an effective service, occupancy should be 80 – 90%, allowing for emergencies – an average of 85%" (RCPsych, 1998b). Quirk and Lelliott (2001) state that "high bed occupancy rates mean that quality of care is compromised. Some people have to be admitted to distant hospitals with subsequent loss of continuity; nurses spend most of their time managing crises rather than giving care". Earlier research by Higgins *et al.* (1999) found that service users were more severely ill in sites with bed occupancy at 100% or more.

Bed occupancy figures are returned by trusts to the Department of Health (DH) (http://www.performance.doh.gov.uk/hospitalactivity). Under the DH category of 'mental illness – other ages short stay (not children and elderly)' their figures for 2002-2003 show average national bed occupancy of 91.4%. Acute bed spaces per 100,000 population are available on Durham mapping by local implementation team but are not available at trust or RDC level (http://www.dur.ac.uk/service.mapping/).

In our survey, we asked trusts to supply the percentage bed occupancy figure calculated over a 12-month period for their acute inpatient wards only for the time period 2003-2004. In total we received annual average bed occupancy percentages for 221 wards. From this we are able to calculate the national average bed occupancy of 100%.

Trust returns on our survey revealed that Eastern region had the highest average bed occupancy at 109% and closer analysis shows that the majority of the 23 wards in the Eastern region had bed occupancies above 100%. The reason for the Eastern region's high bed occupancy is not known and would benefit from further local investigation. London also showed high bed occupancy at 107% (46 wards) and just over two thirds of the wards had occupancy over 100%. High bed occupancy in London is well documented and is also detailed in the Health and Social Care Advisory Service report *Improving the Quality of Psychiatric Inpatient Care in London* (London HAS survey, 2003). In contrast NY&H has the lowest average bed occupancy rate at 91% and a more detailed understanding of how this was achieved by the region could be of enormous value to service providers.

Figure 1   Average bed occupancy rate (221 responses)

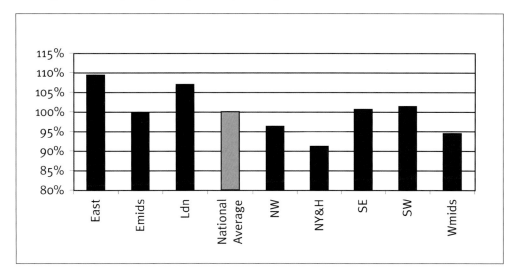

Length of stay   These regional 2002/3 length of stay figures are to be used as a baseline. We took the median length of stay from the HES data. This is calculated by taking the midpoint figure from the length of stay figures for a 12-month period in each region. There were some errors in the HES data such as showing zero days as length of stay as well as invalid dates. We removed these before making our calculations.

We found that the median length of stay varied across the regions from at lowest 38 days (London) to highest at 44 days (East Midlands and South West).

One of the functions of crisis resolution teams is to enable early discharge by providing support at home and therefore the length of stay figures may be one way to start monitoring the impact of such teams.

Diagnoses   To gain an understanding of the diagnoses of service users on acute adult psychiatric wards we have again used the HES data and derived regional percentages. Full details and breakdowns of the diagnostic codes used in the returns to the Department of Health can be found in Chapter V of the *International Statistical Classification of Diseases and Related Health Problems* on the World Health Organisation website (http://www.who.int/classifications/icd/en/) and are attached in Appendix 1. We are using three categories of service user diagnoses: psychoses (such as schizophrenia, bipolar disorder); non-psychoses (such as depression, anxiety, personality disorders); and unknown/non mental health coding. A breakdown of these categories is shown in Appendix 2. The broad category of 'unknown diagnosis' may relate to a coding error or to when a diagnosis has not been made during the admission. We found that non-mental health codes include a wide range of categories varying from problems relating to medical facilities and other health care, and Alzheimer's disease through to asthma. This suggests that while a percentage of non-mental health codes were made accurately, others may have been made as a result of incorrect admission to an acute adult psychiatric ward or errors made in the coding process.

What becomes apparent from Figure 2 is that there is little variation between the regions. London is the exception with a notably lower percentage of service users with non-psychoses, and higher percentages of service users with psychoses and unknown/non mental health coding.

We found from the HES data that 34% of service users were coded as 'psychoses' and across the regions these percentages range from 30% in the Eastern region to 36% in London. Nationally, 49% of service users were coded as 'non-psychoses' and in the regions these percentages range from 42% in London to 52% in the Eastern region.

Nationally, 17% of service users had an 'unknown/non mental health' coding.

If these figures on diagnoses are accurate, then it would suggest that the criteria for admission vary in different parts of the country, most notably in London and Eastern regions.

Figure 2 National breakdown of Finished Consultant Episodes (FCEs) by diagnoses

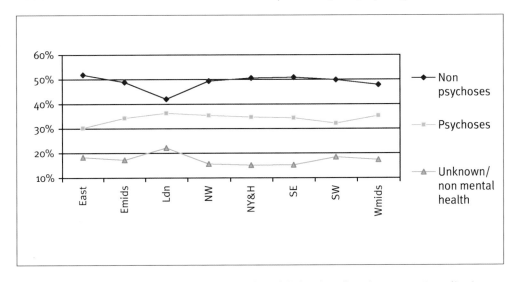

Ethnicity In January 2005, the Department of Health published *Delivering Race Equality in Mental Health Care: An action plan for reform inside and outside services and the Government's response to the independent inquiry into the death of David Bennett* (DH, 2005). The plan sets out what is needed to improve mental health services for those from Black and minority ethnic (BME) communities.

One of the three 'building blocks' outlined is 'better information' and this, in part, relates to the need for more accurate monitoring of ethnicity by trusts. In October 2000, the Department of Health Data Set Change Notice 21/2000 advised that the NHS should use a new set of 16 ethnicity codes. The Department of Health has published training materials and guidance on this (see http://www.statistics. gov.uk/about/ethnic_group_statistics/). These new codes are the same as those used by the Commission for Racial Equality and the Office for National Statistics. The Department of Health states that collecting this ethnicity data is "vital to addressing health inequalities and improvements in public health and commissioning functions" (http://www.dh.gov.uk/PublicationsAndStatistics/ Statistics/StatisticalCollection/fs/en).

On 31 March 2005, The National Mental Health and Ethnicity Census will take place (Mental Health Act Commission [MHAC], Healthcare Commission [HC] and NIMHE). This census will look at the numbers of BME service users, whether "ethnic assessment and record keeping" is in place, whether "culturally capable services" have been implemented and also will "assess disparities" such as in the use of the Mental Health Act. Following the census, interviews with a sample of 2,000 service users will be undertaken in April 2005.

We have taken ethnicity information from the HES data and, where out of date categories have been used, we have converted these to the correct 16 new categories plus a 'not stated' category. From this we have derived regional information.

The 'British, Mixed British' category is the highest percentage across all the regions with the lowest percentage for this category found in London at 54%. Elsewhere, percentages for the 'British, Mixed British' category range from 60% (South East) to 70% (NY&H).

Next highest in all regions was the 'not stated' category. This ranged from 16% (NY&H) to 26% (South East) and highlights the depth of the coding problem. All regions have low percentages of all other ethnic groups (see Appendix 3).

Accurate monitoring of ethnicity is vital if planning and commissioning are to improve and culturally sensitive services are to be offered.

Service users on a section

We asked ward managers to report on the total number of service users on the ward detained under a section of the Mental Health Act at the time they completed the survey. This added up to a national total of 2,371 service users (296 responses). The figures we obtained are a baseline from which wards and trusts will be able to make comparisons in the future particularly when looking at the impact of any changes made to current legislation. Annual figures on the number of service users detained in NHS facilities (including high security psychiatric hospitals) under the Mental Health Act 1983 are presented in the Department of Health statistical bulletin *In-patients formally detained in hospitals under the Mental Health Act 1983 and other legislation 1993-94 to 2003-04* published in December 2004 (http://www.publications.doh.gov.uk/public/sb0422.htm). Our findings relate solely to the acute inpatient ward.

From our survey we found that the majority of service users were being held either on a section 2 or section 3 and numbers for service users held on all other sections was very low. Section 2 is used for admission for assessment up to 28 days whereas section 3 is for treatment up to 6 months.

We have analysed our findings by region and our survey showed that 70% to 84% of service users detained were under section 3 and 14% to 24% were under section 2. Regional use of section 2 and section 3 appears very similar although Eastern region had the highest percentage use of section 2 and the lowest use of section 3. It is not possible to determine why Eastern region's percentages were different and a local review that takes into account bed occupancy, the percentage of service users on wards solely for detoxification, and the availability of other services may be useful.

Escorted leave   The responsible medical officer (RMO), usually a consultant psychiatrist, is the doctor who is in charge of a service user's care. The RMO can grant leave to service users detained under the Mental Health Act and sometimes this leave requires a member of the ward staff to escort the service user. Other service users may be escorted on a voluntary basis. Some ward managers have expressed concerns to us about the impact that escorted leave can have on ward staffing levels, and the need for this to be factored in to calculations for nursing establishments on wards. We asked ward managers how many minutes/hours of escorted leave their ward had on the day that they completed the survey. The national average amounted to 3 hours 57 minutes. However, there were regional differences with East Midlands averaging 1 hour 35 minutes and Eastern region averaging 8 hours 5 minutes. It is not possible to ascertain from the survey if these figures are typical or not.

Figure 3   Average hours spent on escorted leave on day of survey completion (310 responses)

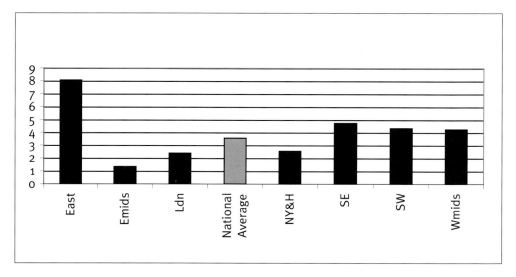

Observations   As well as escorted leave, we asked ward managers how often service users were on one-to-one observations (being 'specialled') or high intensity observations. If a service user's mental state gives cause for increased concern, then high intensity observation may be deemed necessary. This may mean that a member of staff has to stay with a service user continuously. As with escorted leave, one-to-one observations have an impact on staffing pressures on the ward. In a one-day survey carried out by the Mental Health Act Commission, it was found that "nurses spend much of their time engaged in intensive observation of a few patients, but a quarter of wards had no nurse interacting with patients at the time of the visit" (Ford *et al.*, 1998).

Responses to our survey by ward managers reveal that there was considerable variation across the regions. By region, ward managers who reported that high intensity observations occurred frequently ranged from 27% to 61%.

Figure 4   How often does 'Specialling' or high intensity observation occur on the ward? (305 responses)

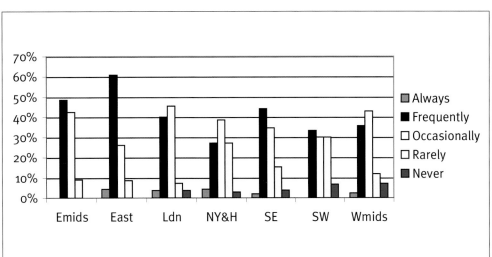

Drugs and alcohol detoxification

The *Mental Health Policy Implementation Guide: Dual diagnosis good practice guide* (Dual diagnosis MH-PIG) states that the term "dual diagnosis covers a broad spectrum of mental health and substance misuse problems that an individual might experience concurrently" (DH, 2002b). Substance misuse includes both drugs and alcohol.

In this survey, we have focused on service users who have been admitted to an acute psychiatric ward solely for detoxification and also on ward managers' perceptions of access to substance misuse services. This survey does not identify the number of beds designated for detoxification and is therefore intended to be a baseline for regional/local use.

We asked ward managers to state how many service users were on the ward solely for detoxification at the time they completed the survey. Figure 5 reveals that there is considerable difference across the regions in both percentages and types of detoxification. The national average of beds used for alcohol detoxification is 2.3% of beds, for drug detoxification 1% and for drug and alcohol detoxification 1%. Eastern and NY&H regions have the highest percentage of beds used for alcohol detoxification (both at 3.2%). Eastern region has the highest percentage of beds used for combined alcohol and drugs detoxification (2.8%). The percentage of beds used solely for drug detoxification is highest in London (1.5%). The reasons for the variation between regions and for the types of detoxification taking place are not known and it is hoped these will act as a trigger for further local investigation.

Figure 5   How many people are currently on the ward solely for detox? (275 responses)

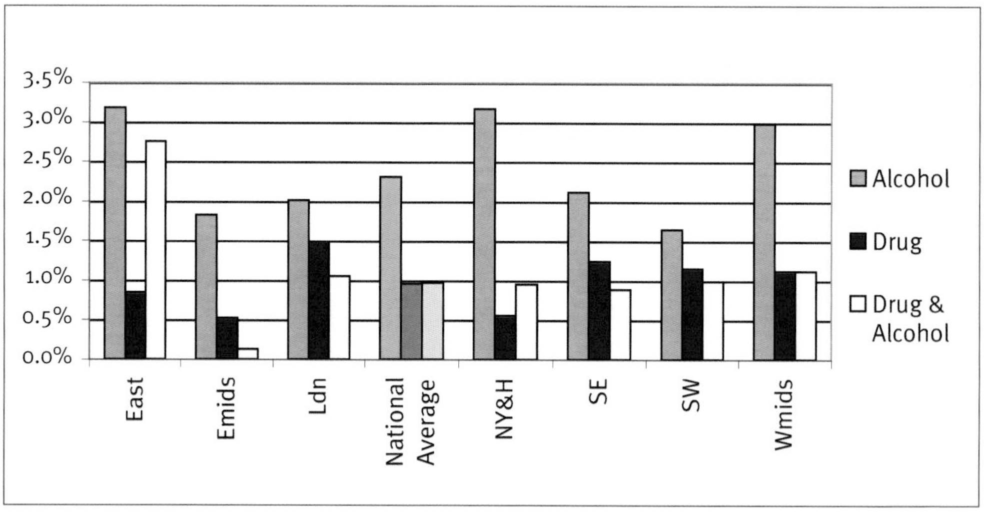

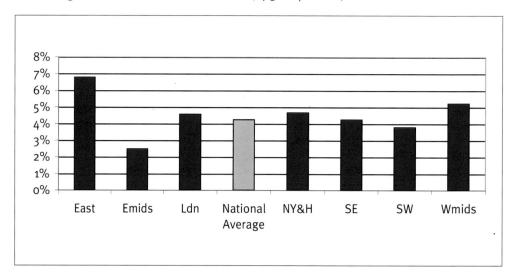

Figure 6 shows an overview of the percentage of acute inpatient beds that were used solely for all types of detoxification. As a percentage of wards that took part in the survey, Eastern region was using the highest proportion of beds for this purpose at 6.8% and East Midlands was using the lowest at 2.5%. From the wards that took part in our survey, we found that nationally a total of 275 beds (4.2%) were being used solely for detoxification at the time of the survey completion.

Figure 6   Percentage of acute beds used for detox (275 responses)

We wanted to ascertain whether ward managers thought there was adequate access to appropriate substance misuse services and nationally 80% of ward managers reported that there was. London, NY&H and South East regions show higher percentages of wards not having adequate access at 31%, 23% and 24% respectively. These are all regions showing high actual numbers of service users on wards solely for detoxification. This survey does not explore the specific issues for ward managers and this would need to be undertaken at a local level.

Figure 7   Do service users with alcohol/drug problems have adequate access to appropriate substance misuse services? (310 responses)

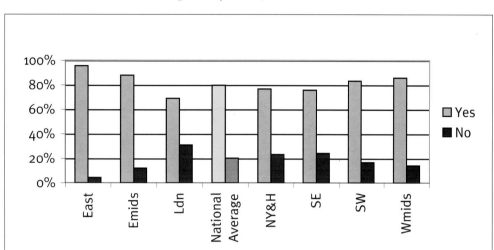

RECOMMENDATIONS

HES returns

❖ The quality of Trust HES returns needs to improve if the HES data is going to inform service provision and monitor improvements.

Bed occupancy and length of stay

❖ Trusts should review bed occupancy levels to check the appropriateness of admissions, as one method of evaluating the impact of community teams and to ensure that staffing levels and skills mix are set at a level adequate to meet demand.

❖ Trusts should use their length of stay figures as one method of evaluating the impact of crisis resolution teams. Lengthy stays need to be monitored, so appropriate action can be taken to alleviate any shortfalls in provision or difficulties in team, service and agency collaboration and communication.

Escorted leave and one-to-one observations

❖ Trusts should audit staff time spent providing escorted leave and observation in order to understand the impact on service users, ward staffing numbers, the use and cost of agency staff and the provision of regular and varied activities on the ward.

Drug/alcohol related

❖ Trusts should review the number of dedicated beds against the actual number of service users brought into wards solely for detoxification. Trusts should then liaise with substance misuse services and drug action teams (DATs) to review local service availability, form a joint agreement on appropriate admission to the adult acute inpatient ward and improve/promote effective communication between ward staff and substance misuse services and DATs.

❖ Trusts should review staffing levels, skill mix, clinical and managerial supervision arrangements and quality of training and safety in view of findings on number of service users brought in solely for detoxification particularly where beds are not ring-fenced for this purpose. The Dual diagnosis MH-PIG (DH, 2002b), *Models of Care for the treatment of drug misusers Part 2* (NTA,

2002) and *Drug Misuse and Dependence: Guidelines on Clinical Management* (DH, 1999b) need to be an integral part of this process.

❖ Strategic health authorities (SHAs) and primary care trust (PCT) commissioners should review the availability of services for people with drug and alcohol problems in the regions identified in the survey as having insufficient services. The Dual diagnosis MH-PIG and *Models of Care for treatment of adult drug misusers Part 1* (NTA, 2002) need to be an integral part of this process.

Ethnicity ❖ Trusts should ensure that staff are adequately informed on how to ask about ethnicity, why ethnicity data is collected and what it is used for. Furthermore they should ensure that the codes used are in line with the Data Set Change Notice 21/2000.

❖ Trusts should involve ACFs and ward managers in looking at ethnic diversity using HES returns, National Mental Health and Ethnicity Census data and the new *Delivering Race Equality* publication (DH, 2005), so that gaps in service provision in acute care can be identified.

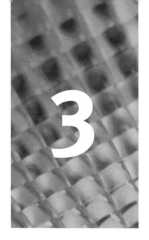

3 Ward purpose

"The purpose of an adult acute psychiatric inpatient service is to provide a high standard of humane treatment and care in a safe and therapeutic setting for service users in the most acute and vulnerable stage of their illness. It should be for the benefit of those service users whose circumstances of acute care needs are such that they cannot at the time be treated and supported appropriately at home or in an alternative, less restrictive residential setting."

Mental Health Policy Implementation Guide:
Adult Acute Inpatient Care Provision (DH, 2002a)

KEY FINDINGS

❖ Almost a quarter of ward managers reported that their wards did not serve their purpose

❖ There were considerable variations in official age ranges for wards but 17% (50 wards) had a lower age limit of 14 years

❖ 87% of ward managers reported having systems in place to regularly monitor the quality of care on the ward

❖ Clinical governance in the trust informed and influenced improvements on 88% of wards

CONTEXT

The *Mental Health Policy Implementation Guide: Adult Acute Inpatient Care Provision* (MH-PIG Adult Acute) sets out the need to reshape the acute inpatient service and includes the role of the acute care forum (ACF) in defining "the therapeutic philosophy and overall service framework of acute inpatient care with specific written service criteria on the purpose and nature of the service provided and the nature of the work, skills, knowledge and attitudes expected of staff" (DH, 2002a). We did not define the ward purpose as the MH-PIG Adult Acute states that there need to be "locally negotiated and agreed operational policies" making one standard definition impossible. Instead ward managers were asked whether they believed that their ward served its purpose. In exploring ward purpose, we also wanted to gain an understanding of how many wards are monitoring the quality of the service they provide and the impact of clinical governance.

The admission of adolescents to adult acute wards has been a subject of longstanding controversy and we wanted to ascertain the age ranges of service users that were accepted on the wards. The *National Service Framework for Children, Young People and Maternity Services: The Mental and Psychological Well-being of Children and Young People* (NSF-Children) states that a marker of good practice is that "child and adolescent mental health services are able to meet the needs of all young people including those aged sixteen and seventeen" (DH, 2004). The NSF-MH states that "if a bed in an adolescent unit cannot be located for a young person, but admission is essential for the safety and welfare of the service user or others, then care may be provided on an adult ward for a short period. As a contingency measure, NHS trusts should identify wards or settings that would be better suited to meet the needs of young people. A protocol must be agreed between the child and adolescent mental health services, and adult services" (DH, 1999a). In their study *Inappropriate admission of young people with mental disorder to adult psychiatric wards and paediatric wards,* Worrall *et al.* (2004) found that a proportion of admissions to both adult and paediatric units was deemed inappropriate and go on to state that their findings "indicate an absolute lack of capacity in child and adolescent inpatient psychiatric units in England and Wales".

At the other end of the scale there may be service users who are older than the specified adult age limit, who require specialist care for older people.

WHAT WE FOUND

Ward purpose   Although 78% of ward managers confirmed that the ward served its purpose as an adult acute inpatient ward, there were still substantial percentages across the regions that gave a negative response. Most notable is the East Midlands region where 13 ward managers (41%) stated that their ward did not serve its purpose. Nationally, a total of 65 ward managers (22%) reported that their ward did not serve its purpose.

Figure 8   Does the ward serve its purpose? (299 responses)

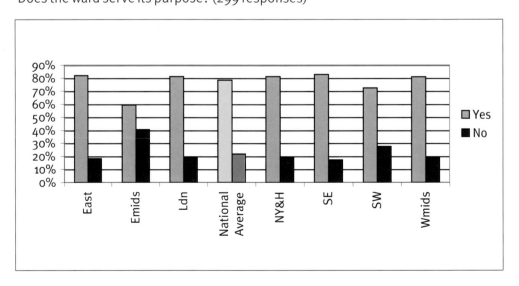

The earlier NW Acute Ward Survey, found that 74% of the wards surveyed had a lower age limit of 16 years (Ryan, 2003). In our survey, we found that official age ranges for acute inpatient wards do vary with some wards having lower age limits between 14 and 17 years and others taking service users who are 65 or over (300 responses). From those that completed this survey question we found that:

❖ 74.4% have an official age range of 18 to 64

❖ 9.3% have an official age range of 14 to 64

❖ 9% have an official age range of 18 to 65+

❖ 7.3% have an official age range of 14 to 65+

We asked whether the wards adhered to their official age ranges and the majority did. We did not explore why wards are not adhering to these ranges and it may be due to lack of local dedicated and appropriate access to services for under 18s and over 65s. There are concerns for areas with high bed occupancy that may already be under pressure if they have to extend their age ranges. Where either adolescents or older people are admitted onto an acute adult ward there are potential concerns about the suitability of the ward environment as well as staff training and the specialist knowledge necessary for their care.

Monitoring quality

87% of ward managers (294 responses) reported that they had systems in place to regularly monitor the quality of care on the ward. London, NY&H, and South West regions had systems in place on over 90% of wards. This survey does not tell us the methods used by wards to ensure a best practice approach to quality monitoring nor whether this is a standard approach across the regions.

Clinical governance informed and influenced improvements on 88% of wards (302 responses) and for NY&H this is the case on 97% of wards. The percentage figure is a little lower for West Midlands and East Midlands both of which are at 78%. The slightly lower figure for East Midlands with regard to clinical governance also reflects a lower figure for quality monitoring on the ward.

RECOMMENDATIONS

Defining ward purpose

❖ Trusts/acute care forums (ACFs) should ensure that all acute inpatient services have a defined purpose as per MH-PIG Adult Acute (DH, 2002a).

❖ PCTs and local authorities should audit admissions so that gaps in service provision or other issues relating to admission criteria can be clearly identified.

Ward age ranges

❖ Trusts/ACFs should understand the implications of ward age restrictions, both official and non-official, in terms of staffing levels and skill mix; supervision and training needs; environment; safety; and service user needs.

❖ PCTs and local authorities need to review service provision for adolescents and older people in order to stop the admission of adolescents and inappropriate admissions of older people to adult wards.

Quality monitoring

❖ Trust clinical governance leads and ACFs, in collaboration with PCT and SHA leads, should review the monitoring of quality in wards across regions and work towards increasing shared quality measures.

❖ ACFs/clinical governance leads should review the role of clinical governance within trusts, in particular to assess how information is both shared and utilised to improve service user safety and the quality of services.

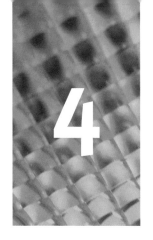

4 Information for service users

"The first 72 hours seem particularly important in an individual's admission, requiring orientation, guidance, information, engagement, and reassurance."

Mental Health Policy Implementation Guide:
Adult Acute Inpatient Care Provision (DH, 2002a)

KEY FINDINGS

❖ 83% of ward managers reported that their wards provided over 50% of the recommended information for service users

❖ Gaps in information related mainly to provision of a floor plan for the ward, picture board of ward staff and a code of conduct that included what was expected of all service users on the ward

❖ 68% of ward managers reported that they used over 50% of user/carer involvement methods

❖ 97% of ward managers confirmed that they provided information to service users and carers on how to make complaints

CONTEXT

The importance of providing sufficient information to service users admitted to the ward has long been known. Rose (2001) found that "access to good information is significantly associated with how satisfied users say they are with mental health services as a whole". However, the report *Acute Problems* identified that service users and staff on the whole had very different views about the provision of information about illnesses and treatments given (SCMH, 1998). The National Audit of Violence being conducted by the Royal College of Psychiatrists (2003 – 2005) has asked service users from a range of wards and units, including acute inpatient wards, about satisfaction with the provision of a variety of types of information such as how the ward was run; decisions about care and support, why they were on the unit and medication and treatments. Their initial findings show that a quarter or more of those surveyed still feel that they are not being given sufficient information (Royal College of Psychiatrists, unpublished).

The Department of Health has a range of guidance and templates for service user information leaflets specifically aimed at mental health services and these can be found on its website under "good practice in patient care and improving the patient experience" (http://www.dh.gov.uk/PolicyAndGuidance/OrganisationPolicy/PatientAndPublicInvolvement). Mind has recently made available a publication designed to help with this admission process entitled *How to cope with hospital admission* (Campbell, 2004).

Although there is still scope for further improvement, the findings in this report are encouraging and show that much has been done to improve provision of information to service users and carers.

WHAT WE FOUND

Provision of information for service users

The *Mental Health Policy Implementation Guide: Adult Acute Inpatient Care Provision* (MH-PIG Adult Acute) makes very specific reference to a range of information that wards should provide as good practice on reception and service orientation to service users (DH, 2002a). Ward managers were asked in our survey whether their wards provided each of the 15 recommended items. Responses were returned from all wards. We found that 83% of all ward managers reported that their wards provided over 50% of the recommended items. Seven of these wards (2%) provided the full range of information. Those seven wards were not all located within the same region, suggesting small pockets of excellent practice. There were, however, 52 wards (17%) in the country providing less than 50% of the recommended information and two wards that worryingly reported providing none of the recommended information.

Table 3   Information for service users

Service user information	Provided
Explanatory information on illness	88%
Clear policy on contact with relatives and friends and visiting times	87%
A service user handbook/guide on what is available in the ward and how to access it	85%
Explanatory information on symptoms	85%
Good signage	84%
Clear policy on leave	75%
Explanatory information on courses of treatment	74%
Explanatory information on trust services	72%
Clear policy on access to telephones	72%
Clear policy on access	65%
Code of conduct – including what to expect from staff	64%
A service user orientation checklist as part of care plan	64%

Code of conduct – including what to expect of all service users on the ward	55%
A floor plan/map of the ward and the unit	34%
A picture board of ward staff, prominently displayed	26%

Service user/ carer involvement

Rose (2001) states that "the measurement of the extent of user involvement at all levels should be the extent to which users themselves feel involved" and that "users should be at the centre of the monitoring and evaluation of mental health services". The Commission for Health Improvement (now Healthcare Commission) 2003 report *What CHI has found in mental health trusts* found "examples where user involvement is embedded in the principles and practice of trusts at every level" but it was also noted that "user involvement is still inconsistent in many areas".

Wards were asked about the types of methods used to ensure user or carer involvement. The majority of wards (68%) used between 50% and 99% of the methods listed and a further seven ward managers (2%) reported that they used all of the listed methods of user/carer involvement. However, there remain 98 wards (32%) that used less than 50% of the methods listed. Table 4 shows the overall national percentages.

Table 4   Service user/carer involvement

Service user/carer involvement	Provided
Community meetings	83%
Acute Care Forum	82%
Patient Advice and Liaison Service (PALS)	79%
Independent advocacy	65%
Satisfaction questionnaire	53%
Trust funded/staffed advocacy	49%
Patient Councils	44%
User audit	41%
User-focused monitoring	39%

We then asked the separate question of whether service users and carers were informed as to how they could make complaints. A total of 302 ward managers (97%) stated that they did provide this information to service users and carers.

From the data collected, we are able to see that provision of information to service users is variable even within the same trusts. This could indicate that there is no standard approach or standard documentation within trusts to bring practice into line with the policy implementation guide recommendations.

It is encouraging that the majority of wards are now providing 50% or more of the recommended information, but this report identifies the need for some further work in this area.

RECOMMENDATIONS

Positive practice and information sharing

❖ Acute care forums (ACFs) should provide clarification to wards on what constitutes positive practice and promote implementation of the policy guidance and DH examples of good practice/templates.

❖ Local authorities, ACFs, trusts and RDCs should work together in sharing information and disseminating good practice.

Evaluation and audit

❖ Trusts should involve service users and carers in the evaluation of ward reception and orientation in order to identify good practice and areas for improvement.

❖ Trusts should undertake evaluations/audits to ensure staff and service user/carer perceptions match.

❖ Trusts should organise internal/external audits of both the quality of information provided to service users and carers and the dissemination of information to service users and carers.

On the wards

❖ Ward managers should ensure that all service users are provided with information regardless of how many times they have previously been admitted.

❖ Ward managers should have a designated person to ensure information packs are kept up-to-date and in stock, and picture boards of staff are kept up-to-date etc.

❖ Ward managers should ensure that there is a designated person on the shift to greet and provide information to service users (and carers, relatives, friends) upon arrival e.g. housekeeper, member of ward staff, voluntary worker etc.

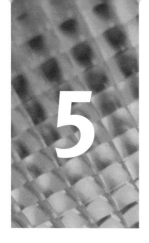

5 Ward staffing

"Too many inpatient wards do not have the levels of staff and skills available to deliver the required standard of care and as such the quality of the worklife of the inpatient staff is constantly compromised."

Mental Health Policy Implementation Guide: Adult Acute Inpatient Care Provision (DH,2002a)

KEY FINDINGS

❖ 52% of wards had a lead consultant

❖ 87% of wards were run by a ward manager or nurse above an F grade

❖ 41% of ward managers reported that they had frequently undertaken bed management outside their own ward

❖ The national average vacancy rate for qualified nurses was 13% and was as high as 22% in London at the time of the survey

❖ The national average vacancy rate for health care assistants was 2.7% at the time of the survey

❖ 26% of ward managers reported that staff had regularly worked unpaid overtime in the previous 12 months

❖ The national average combined bank and agency usage (all grades) per week per ward was 151.6 hours which equates to 4.04 whole time equivalents

❖ 88% of wards had administrative support

❖ 26% of ward managers reported that staff had left to join community teams in the previous 12 months

CONTEXT

The difficulties in staffing acute inpatient units and calculating optimal staffing levels and skill mix are not new. The report *What CHI has found in mental health trusts,* states that in "inpatient areas there are particular concerns about staffing levels, skill mix, the use of locum, bank and agency staff and the impact of low staffing levels on staff safety" (Healthcare Commission, 2003) and these concerns are echoed in Mind's *Ward Watch* campaign report published in 2004. The specific staffing problems for the London region have been highlighted in the London HAS

Report (2003) as well as in the report by the King's Fund *London's Mental Health Workforce: A review of recent developments* (Genkeer *et al.,* 2003).

Lack of resources makes it hard to implement and sustain change and CHI reported that meeting the "challenges set out in the national service framework are dependent on these capacity issues being resolved" (Healthcare Commission, 2003). These changes are having an impact on the nurse role with an "increased expectation on them in terms of care delivery, using evidence based treatments, carrying out audit, research, practice development, maintaining notes, providing a resource for carers and reflecting and improving on their practice" (HAS, 2003).

Colleagues in the Joint Workforce Support Unit, a joint unit between SCMH and NIMHE, carried out work in early 2004 looking at overall consultant psychiatrist vacancies, difficulties in recruitment, the use of locums and the impact for staff teams of difficulties in recruiting (due to be published 2005). Their survey did not specify acute inpatients but they did look at adult services as a whole and they found almost 1,500 posts of which over 175 were vacant in England. In 2003, the average number of candidates applying for General Adult posts was only 1.5 per advertised vacancy and only 76% of advertised vacancies were successfully filled (Hoadley *et al.,* unpublished).

We wanted to find out more about multidisciplinary input onto acute inpatient wards including differences between funded and actual establishments and, for nurses, agency and bank usage. Trusts were able to provide information on numbers of nurses, health care assistants, occupational therapists (OTs), OT assistants and housekeepers, but it soon became clear there were problems in providing the same information about other professional groups such as psychiatrists, psychologists, art therapists, support time recovery workers, activity workers and others. These difficulties are largely due to the way services are configured with these staff groups often working across inpatient, community and outpatient settings. It would also seem that there are some difficulties with how to define posts that do not fall under distinct categories. The King's Fund report recognises these problems and recommends that "Workforce Development Confederations should carry responsibility for compiling robust data specifically relating to the mental health workforce" which could then inform workforce planning and design (Genkeer *et al.,* 2003). In essence this lack of data leaves the total multidisciplinary staff input into acute inpatient wards unknown.

In addition, we asked ward managers about a range of issues including numbers of ward reviews, administrative support, bed management, paid and unpaid overtime, sickness and absence, disciplinary action, recruitment and information on where staff had moved on to when leaving their ward.

WHAT WE FOUND

**Psychiatrists
– Lead consultant**

The *Mental Health Policy Implementation Guide: Adult Acute Inpatient Care Provision* (MH-PIG Adult Acute) states that "each inpatient ward/service must have its own dedicated lead consultant psychiatrist who can provide expert input into key matters of inpatient service delivery, staff support and supervision, and overall acute care service co-ordination" (DH, 2002a).

There are still a number of wards throughout the country that do not have a lead consultant. In our survey we found that 144 wards (48%) do not have a lead consultant. The highest numbers of wards with lead consultants are found in Eastern region and in London at 70% and 79% respectively.

Figure 9   Wards with dedicated lead consultant (303 responses)

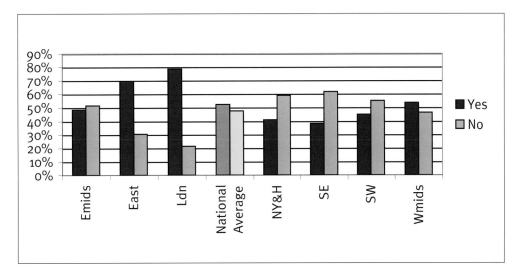

**Use of beds
and ward reviews**

Anecdotally, some ward managers expressed concerns about the number of consultants using beds on their wards and the consequent increase in ward reviews/rounds. The NW Acute Ward Survey revealed that the average number of ward reviews being carried out per week was 4.6 (Ryan, 2003). The London HAS report (2003) found that it was not unusual "to find large inpatient wards having ward or management rounds on most days of the week excluding weekends". At least one qualified nurse will usually need to take part in the review. On wards with only one or two qualified nurses per shift or mainly agency and bank staff this can affect the leadership of the ward as well as ward activities.

Our survey revealed that the number of consultants who have allocated beds on the wards varies across the regions from 2.7 to 3.6. However, the actual number of consultants using beds on the wards shows a very different picture with numbers ranging from 4.3 to 6.7 across the regions. From the survey replies we received from Eastern region, it seems that they had the highest number of consultant psychiatrists actually using beds on the wards. With high numbers of consultants, this can potentially lead to an increase in the number of ward reviews per week. Our survey shows that these average out to between 4.1 and 5 across the regions. It is not surprising to see that Eastern region has the highest average number of ward reviews per week.

Figure 10   Average no. of consultants and ward reviews (310 responses)

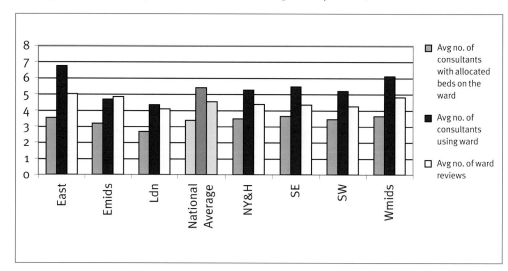

Ward managers   The MH-PIG Adult Acute states that a "lack of leadership focus on inpatient service structure, delivery and system co-ordination exacerbates over-occupancy and over pressurised ward environments thus prompting a more custodial and less engaging and therapeutic model of inpatient care" (DH, 2002a).

The majority of ward managers are usually H or G grade nurses but there are some units where the ward manager role is a non-nursing post. We wanted to find out how many wards had a ward manager or nurse above F grade. Our survey responses show that 39 (13%) wards had neither a ward manager nor a nurse above F Grade at the time of survey. The regional breakdown is listed in Table 5.

Table 5   Regional breakdown of ward manager grades

RDC	Wards with no manager or nurse above F grade	Total number of survey responses to this question	% Wards with no manager or nurse above F grade
East	4	27	15%
Emids	1	13	8%
Ldn	10	76	13%
NY&H	4	59	7%
NW	13	30	43%
SE	3	48	6%
SW	0	18	0%
Wmids	4	32	13%
Totals	**39**	**303**	**13%**

This national percentage is high and the lack of ward managers needs urgent review particularly in the North West where almost half of the wards that were included in the survey are without a nurse above an F grade. This finding, alongside the shortfall in lead consultants for the wards, suggests that there are areas running with insufficient leadership.

Bed management   As well as the management of their own wards, ward managers may be expected to undertake bed management outside their own ward. The picture by region shows considerable variation in how frequently this occurs. Nationally, 126 ward managers (41%) reported that they frequently undertook bed management outside their ward. Bed management outside the ward was high for ward managers in the Eastern (61%), London and West Midlands regions (both 55%). Noting that nationally 99 ward managers reported never or only rarely having had to do this and 82 sometimes had to do this, this reveals a potential disparity in role expectation/ requirement. It may be that in some areas the modern matron has taken over this role or that there is a specific bed manager for the hospital. On wards, particularly where the ward manager is counted in the staffing numbers for the shift, this may have an important impact on the staffing levels of the shift and/or leadership of the ward.

Figure 11   How often does the ward manager take responsibility for bed management outside of their own ward? (307 responses)

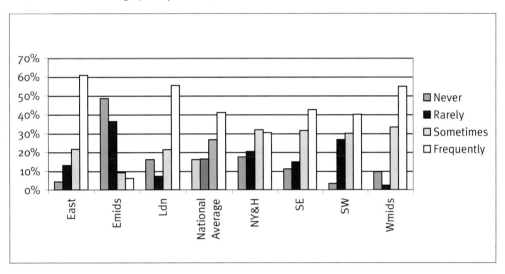

Staff sickness rates   The results of the NHS Sickness and Absence Survey 2003 show that in 'Mental Health and Community', the average sickness and absence rate is 5.5%. This contrasts with the NHS as whole, which has an average sickness rate of 4.7% (http://www.publications.doh.gov.uk/public/sicknessabsence2003.htm).

We found from our staffing survey that for the time period of 2003 to 2004, the average national sickness on acute inpatients wards was 6.8% (227 responses). This suggests that inpatient wards are running at higher levels of sickness than other parts of mental health and community services and considerably higher than the average for the NHS as a whole. This level of sickness and absence will affect the continuity of care for service users and is likely to increase stress and/or workload for remaining staff, as well as incurring higher costs for bank and agency nurse cover.

Higgins *et al.* (1999) found that short-term staff sickness rose on some wards as more severely ill service users were admitted and that nurses admitted to having taken occasional sick days as "owing to the demanding nature of their current workload, recourse to such coping strategies was necessary but taken with great reluctance". The Commission for Health Improvement found that "many permanent staff are working excessive hours, and ...found weaknesses in the systems to monitor staff working hours" (Healthcare Commission, 2003). This backs up the recommendations of Higgins *et al.* (1999) that "senior managers should examine the pattern and levels of staff sickness and overtime to ascertain the extent of the problem. Excessive overtime and sickness seem to be influenced by patient dependency, nursing workload, nursing establishment and grade mix".

Disciplinary action

Some 77 ward managers (26%) reported that they had taken disciplinary action against a member of staff in the previous 12 months (this does not show the numbers of incidents of disciplinary action within each ward). Across the regions the numbers ranged from 4 ward managers (16%) at lowest in the East Midlands to 19 ward managers (35%) at highest in the South East. We did not explore the reasons for this disciplinary action as part our survey and this would need to be undertaken as a part of a local review by human resource departments.

Figure 12   Wards where disciplinary action was taken against a member of staff in the previous 12 months (296 responses)

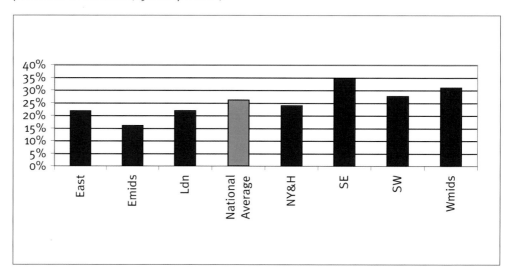

Nursing staff

There is no easy formulation for working out the correct numbers of nurses and health care assistants for wards. Many factors need to be taken into account such as number of beds, bed occupancy, staff timeout (training, supervision, annual leave, sickness, maternity leave), the severity of illness and mix of diagnoses of the service users including one-to-one observations and escorted leave, levels of staff expertise and skills, supernumerary or otherwise status of the ward manager, input from disciplines such as OTs and psychologists, administrative support and others. All these factors will lead to variation across wards, trusts and regions and this may be one reason why we see such variation in funded establishments. However, it may also be due to a lack of national guidance on how to set establishments which has led to a number of *ad hoc* and historical methods being used to calculate staffing levels.

We wanted to find out about the numbers of nursing and health care assistant staff per bed to give a baseline understanding of existing staffing numbers. The figures obtained were part of our staffing survey completed by trusts. As the London HAS report (2003) points out one of the dangers of such benchmarking is the "possible assumption that establishments are accepted as the range for inpatient wards" when it is possible that the figures "could be generally too low for the high standards set out in the Policy Implementation Guide". It is with this same caution that we present the analysis of nursing staff to bed ratios.

The qualified nursing staff to bed ratio was calculated excluding any agency or bank staff and taken from figures gathered in the staffing survey. The national average number of funded qualified nurses per bed is 0.74 whole time equivalent (WTE) and the actual number is 0.64 WTE. If, for example, one took a 16-bedded ward, this would mean a shortfall of 1.6 WTE. At a regional level the biggest difference between funded and actual is found in London, where the funded is 0.78 WTE and the actual is 0.60 WTE.

Figure 13   Average qualified nurses per bed ratio (268 responses)

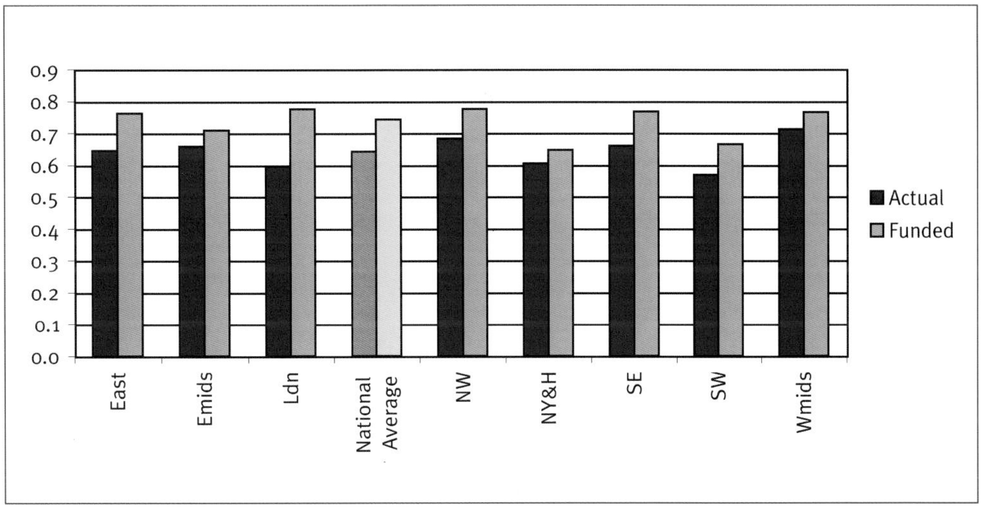

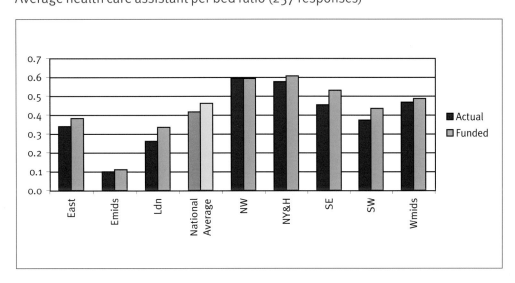

Health care assistant numbers averaged at 0.46 WTE funded and 0.42 WTE actual. This works out as a national average to a shortfall of 0.04 WTE which on the example of a 16-bedded ward equates to 0.64 WTE.

Figure 14   Average health care assistant per bed ratio (257 responses)

Looking at the combined figures of health care assistants and qualified nurses, the national average funded is 1.19 WTE and the actual is 1.06 WTE showing a shortfall of 0.13 WTE per bed. There are no regions where the actual is meeting the funded establishment. Taking these national averages, this would mean that on the example of a 16-bedded ward there would be a shortfall of 2.08 WTE. However, the caveat here is that it is not known whether the funded establishments are set to meet the current and/or new demands of the service.

Figure 15   Average health care assistant and qualified nurse per bed ratio (268 responses)

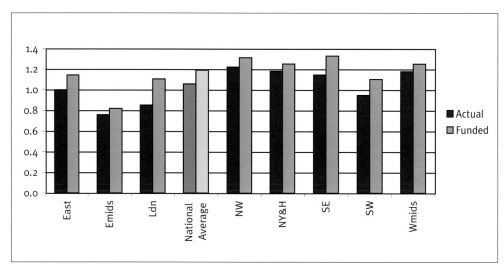

Unfilled nursing and health care assistant posts

In the survey we asked trusts to report back on vacancy rates as defined by the National Workforce Dataset Version 1.0, October 2003. However, only two trusts reported back on vacancy rates as defined and this amounted to data for 17 (6%) wards. Given the small numbers of trusts that reported staff vacancies, it was decided that the percentage of unfilled posts should be calculated using the following formula: funded posts minus staff in post converted to a percentage. The funded posts and staff in post figures were taken from our staffing survey completed by trusts.

We found that nationally there was a 13% average vacancy rate for qualified nurses. We found the highest percentage vacancy rate was in London at 22%. The *London's Mental Health Workforce* report states that "despite being a training ground for health care professionals from across the UK and abroad, London struggles to retain staff within a few years of qualification, due to high living costs" (Genkeer *et al.* 2003).

Figure 16   Unfilled qualified nursing posts (292 responses)

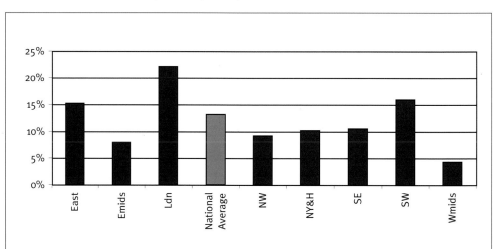

The average vacancy rate for health care assistants was 2.7%. In the Eastern and NY&H regions, the actual number of health care assistants exceeded the funded establishment. The percentage differences were very similar in both regions to the shortfall for qualified nurses. This may indicate that health care assistants were being recruited to cover the shortfall of qualified nurses and to increase numbers per bed. Alternatively it may indicate that the funded health care assistant posts were set too low.

Figure 17   Unfilled health care assistant posts (293 responses)

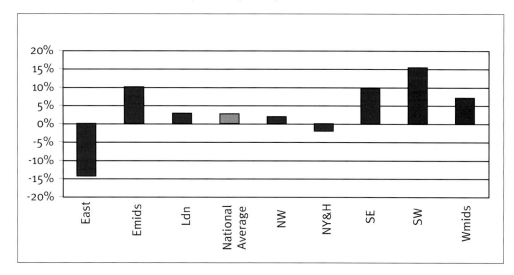

As some wards may operate a degree of flexibility in the skill mix they use depending on local recruitment difficulties, we have also explored the combined nursing and health care assistant unfilled posts. The national average vacancy rate for the combined posts was 12% and this was highest in London where it averaged 21%.

Figure 18   Unfilled qualified nursing and health care assistant posts (292 responses)

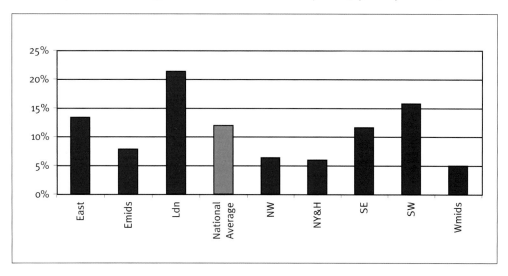

Overtime by ward staff   We asked ward managers how often staff had worked unpaid overtime in the previous 12 months and 78 (26%) responded that their staff had regularly carried out unpaid overtime. This occurred more in the Eastern region than elsewhere with 39% of ward managers having reported that staff regularly worked unpaid overtime. We do not know from this survey if staff were able to take time off in lieu during less busy periods. Nationally, a further 64 ward managers reported that their staff occasionally worked unpaid overtime. In contrast, 101 ward managers reported that staff never worked unpaid overtime with a further 62 stating this rarely happened.

Figure 19   How often have staff worked unpaid overtime on the ward in the past 12 months?
(305 responses)

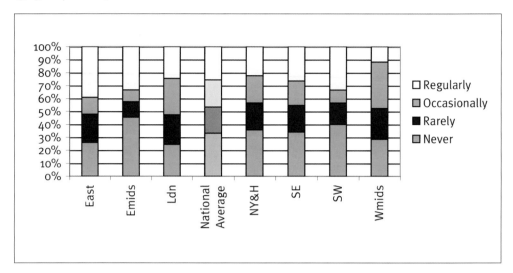

Paid overtime happens much more, with 178 managers (58%) reporting that their staff regularly carried out paid overtime. This occurs most frequently in the East Midlands (73%) and the South East (70%). From our results we are unable to distinguish between true overtime and staff doing extra hours on their own ward via the bank. Nationally, a further 57 wards stated that this had happened occasionally in the previous 12 months. Interestingly, there is a small percentage of wards in each region where staff had never worked paid overtime in the previous 12 months. These differences within regions may be accounted for by local policies on overtime.

Figure 20   How often have staff worked paid overtime on the ward in the past 12 months? (305 responses)

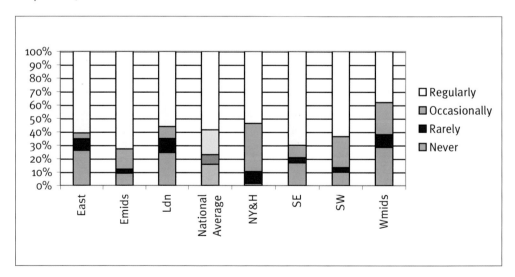

Agency and bank staff   We wanted to gain a picture of agency and bank usage across the country. We asked ward managers to let us know how many hours of agency and bank staff usage there had been on the ward during the previous week, for both qualified and unqualified staff.

The national average for agency staff hours per week per ward was 46.5 hours. A permanent member of the ward team would normally work 37.5 hours so this equates to 1.24 whole time equivalent (WTE). It should be noted that there was considerable variation not only across the regions but also within regions, with some wards showing high agency usage and others reporting that they had only used bank staff. From the survey responses we have received, the highest average percentages for the use of agency staff were found in the South East and London.

Figure 21   Weekly average agency staff hours per ward (266 responses)

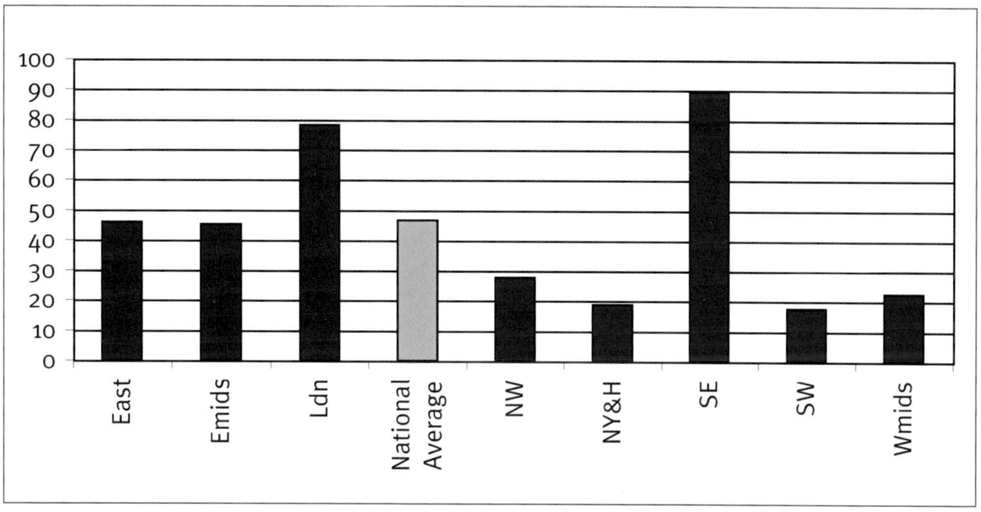

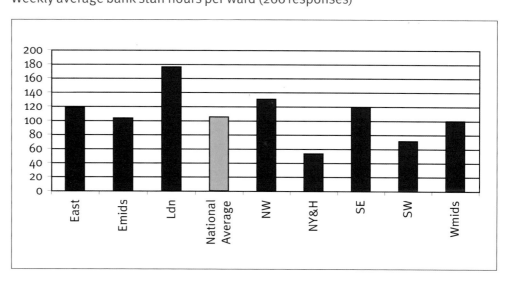

Wards would be expected to use bank staff rather than agency staff where possible both to reduce costs and to have staff that are familiar with the hospital. Bank staff usage was accordingly higher at a national average of 105 hours per week. This equated to 2.8 WTE. Again, we can see regional variation with London, the North West, South East and Eastern region using the largest amounts.

Figure 22   Weekly average bank staff hours per ward (266 responses)

To see the overall picture, we combined agency and bank usage and found that the national average per ward was 151.6 hours and this equated to 4.04 WTE per ward as a national average. It is clear that London and the South East used the highest combined amounts of agency and bank staff with 254 hours (6.8 WTE) and 209 hours (5.6 WTE) respectively.

Figure 23 Weekly average agency and bank staff hours per ward (266 responses)

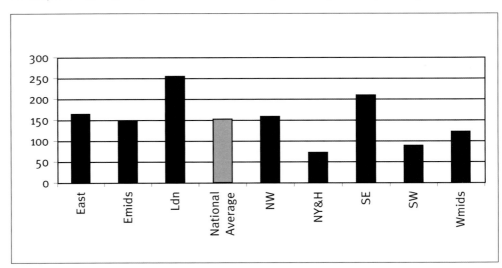

Apart from the obvious issue of vacancies, it remains unclear whether the funded establishments are set too low to meet the requirements of the service, so exacerbating the ongoing need for agency and bank staff. We are not able to state whether this bank and agency usage fills the unfilled posts. The bank and agency figure is based only on one week's usage and would need to be monitored over time to see if it covers the vacancies. In order to gain a deeper understanding more work needs to be undertaken to explore these findings at regional and trust level. However, we can see that London had the highest agency and bank usage, but it also had the largest difference between funded and actual establishment. There was a similar pattern for the South East.

Occupational therapists Occupational therapists (OTs) have an important role in involving service users in therapeutic activity and interaction. As with nursing staff and health care assistants there are no specific recommended establishment figures for OTs and OT assistants. It is therefore unclear what drives the differences in funded establishments across the regions. Recruitment may be one issue and the College of Occupational Therapists (COT) is preparing a mental health strategy which will look at recruitment and retention, to be published in 2005. From our survey, it is not possible to gauge whether funded establishments are set at an appropriate level to provide the required standard of care. The national average shows that both the actual and funded establishments are at 0.03 OTs per bed (202 responses). If we use the example again of a 16-bedded ward this would equate to 0.5 WTE for the ward.

OT assistants The national average also shows that as for qualified OTs there is no difference between the funded and actual establishments. There are on average 0.014 OT assistants per bed (202 responses) and using the example of a 16-bedded ward this equates to 0.2 WTE for the ward.

Administrative support on the ward The MH-PIG Adult Acute states that "each ward should have specific ward based clerical/administrative support covering the 24-hour operation of the ward" (DH, 2002a). Ward clerks are the group who undertake the bulk of ward-based administrative support. We wanted to find out how much administrative support in terms of hours per week wards were getting and whether this was sustained when the administrative person was on leave etc. There was considerable variation between the regions on the number of hours of administrative support wards were receiving and also considerable variation within regions. In total, 37 wards (12%) around the country reported receiving no administrative support. Where wards have no support it is likely that health care assistants and qualified nurses will be undertaking the administrative tasks that are carried out by ward clerks elsewhere.

Figure 24   How many hours dedicated ward-based admin. support does your ward currently have? (305 responses)

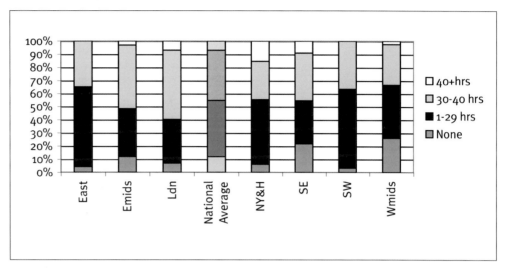

In terms of holiday cover etc. for admin. support staff, 42% of wards reported never having cover and a further 10% reported rarely having cover. Those not receiving cover are most notable in the East Midlands, South East and Eastern regions. Only 8% of wards reported always receiving cover and a further 23% usually receive cover.

Figure 25   Is admin./clerical cover provided when staff go on holiday etc.? (296 responses)

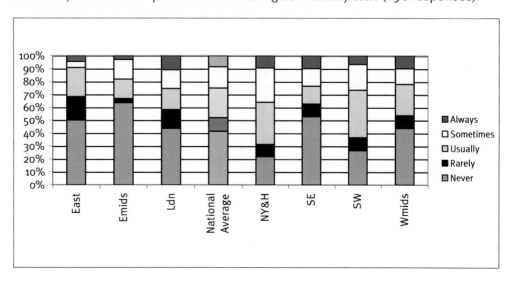

On wards with high numbers of bank and agency staff it is potentially the regular staff, who are familiar with the administrative processes and service users, who are most likely to cover the ward clerk's role.

Housekeepers

The NHS Plan states that "half of all hospitals will have new 'ward housekeepers' in place by 2004" (DH, 2000a) and by September 2003 NHS Estates reported that 40% of all hospitals had introduced housekeeping services. Ward housekeepers are responsible to ward managers and are ward based. They carry out a range of non-clinical work such as ensuring the ward is clean, equipment is maintained, service users receive good quality food and drink, service user privacy and dignity is protected, and they undertake other service user-focused work. One of the aims of having a housekeeper role is to "leave the nursing staff free to do the job they were trained for – nursing patients back to health" (http://www.nhsestates.gov. uk/patient_environment/content/ward_housekeeping.html). More details of the role can be found in the NHS Estates 2001 publication *Housekeeping: A first guide to new, modern and dependable ward housekeeping services in the NHS* (www. nhsestates.gov.uk/download/ward_housekeeping/housekeeping.pdf).

We wanted to find out what was happening on the acute inpatient ward in mental health services. Trusts at present provide quarterly returns to NHS Estates on the numbers of housekeepers they have. However, it appears from the returns on our staffing survey that there were issues around the definition of housekeepers and trusts appear in some instances to have provided information on domestic staff or staff covering aspects of the housekeeper role rather than specifically on housekeepers. For this reason, it is very likely that the figure of 26% (303 responses) of wards that reported having housekeepers is overstated. Trusts that completed the survey in the East Midlands and North West regions reported not having any housekeepers on their acute inpatient wards.

Nursing population, recruitment and staff movement

The Office for National Statistics report on the 2001 Census showed that the non-White population "is concentrated in the large urban centres" and that "nearly half (45%) lived in the London region in 2001, where they comprised 29% of all residents" (http://www.statistics.gov.uk). Figures on the geographical distribution of asylum seekers and refugees have not been made available but it is feasible that a similar pattern would be found. Given the potential ethnic diversity in some parts of London, it may be harder to ensure that the nursing population reflects the general population.

50% of ward managers reported that specific initiatives had taken place to encourage employment of nursing staff to reflect the ethnic profile of the catchment area population. This is particularly marked in the South East where 32 ward managers (59%) reported this was the case. Nationally, 28% of ward managers reported being unsure whether specific initiatives had taken place and these wards were across all regions.

Figure 26   Have specific initiatives taken place to encourage employment of nursing staff to reflect the ethnic profile of the population? (298 responses)

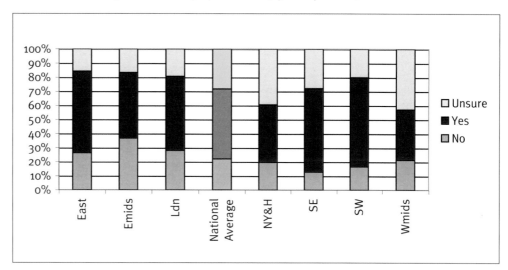

To inform our understanding of recruitment, ward managers were asked where they had recruited staff from in the previous 12 months. The bulk of nursing staff recruited were newly qualified nurses with a total of 282 ward managers reporting this. Second highest was recruitment of staff from other acute inpatient NHS wards and then bank and agency with 147 and 136 managers respectively reporting these. There is some drift from community into acute wards and other small areas of recruitment from return to nursing, the private sector and other.

Figure 27   Where have nursing staff been recruited from in the past 12 months? (310 responses)

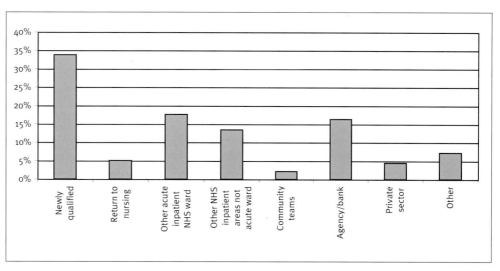

We wanted to understand the staff movement between trusts, regions and from overseas in terms of recruitment and we discovered that most of the recruitment comes from within the trust with 207 ward managers reporting this. The next highest area of recruitment was from within the region with lower numbers having reported that they had recruited from outside the region and/or from overseas. From other SCMH work on staff recruitment and movement it has been identified that in many cases labour markets for professional staff are 'sub-regional'; staff movement between employers is restricted by an individual's home address. Few staff are moving house to change their job in mental health services.

Figure 28 In the past 12 months, from where geographically have you recruited nursing staff? (310 responses)

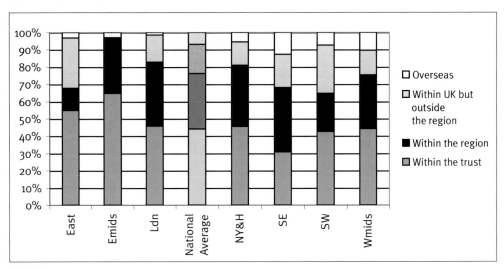

The MH-PIG Adult Acute states that "whereas community mental health nurses are properly recognised as specialists, there is little recognition of the specialist expertise and skills, knowledge and attitudes required of nurses working in inpatient services" (DH, 2002a) and this may be driving the shift of ward staff into community services. Just over a quarter of all managers (26%) reported that staff had left the wards to join community teams in the previous 12 months (see Figure 29). This survey does not tell us how many staff from each ward moved from acute inpatient care into the community. It does however provide evidence of the drain from acute inpatient care into the community and reveals some of the impact of setting up new community teams in a limited staffing pool.

Figure 29 Which community teams have qualified staff moved on to from the ward in the past 12 months? (310 responses)

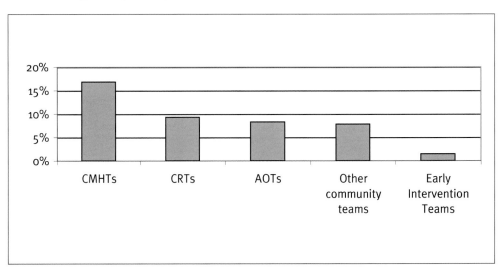

The next largest move reported by ward managers is staff leaving their ward to work elsewhere in the NHS. In total, 14% of ward managers reported staff had moved to other NHS trusts with smaller numbers going on to other wards within the trust or going into management.

Figure 30   Where within the NHS have qualified staff moved on to from the ward in the past 12 months? (310 responses)

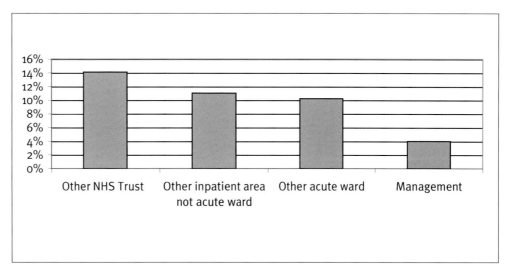

The remaining staff that had left the ward were reported by ward managers to have gone into full time education, education posts, other statutory sectors, private and voluntary sectors. A total of 6.7% ward managers (59) reported that nurses from their ward had left nursing altogether but this would also include nurses who were retiring.

Figure 31   Where outside the NHS have qualified staff moved on to from the ward in the past 12 months? (310 responses)

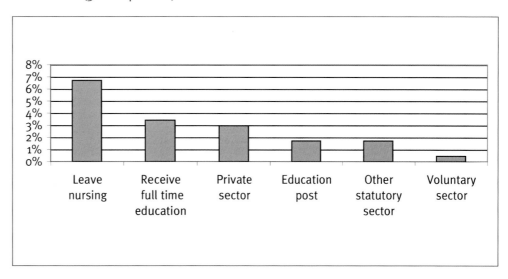

RECOMMENDATIONS

The survey showed acute inpatient services under strain across the country with widespread difficulties regarding adequate staffing. From the results there are a number of key recommendations:

Reviewing staffing levels, skill mix

❖ PCTs, SHAs and trusts should review the role of inpatient services and the skills, roles and overall staffing required for these services. Consideration of the suggestions in the Adult Acute MH-PIG relating to single management of acute care services and a whole systems approach should be taken (see community teams section recommendations).

❖ NIMHE, in association with the National Mental Health Partnership Boards and professional bodies, should work collaboratively to develop guidelines to inform appropriate staffing levels and skill mix.

❖ Trusts in the interim should review their funded establishments for all staff groups and ensure that all factors that will affect required staffing numbers are taken into consideration. Factors may include special observation, sickness and absence, training, supervision, escorts and therapeutic observation and engagement.

❖ Trusts should explore all the reasons for overtime, bank and agency use on wards. As part of this review, trusts should explore why permanent staff who wish to work some additional hours may be opting to work for agencies rather than on the bank (e.g. not being paid their usual grade working on the bank).

Leadership

❖ Trusts should look at the leadership roles and training of acute inpatient staff focusing on provision of lead consultants and ward managers and the grading and skills of staff in leadership roles.

❖ Trusts/ACFs should explore the issue of ward reviews and bed management to see if there are any changes in practice that would be beneficial to service users and the running of the ward.

Recruitment and retention

❖ Workforce organisations/higher education institutions/NIMHE should assist trusts in developing career pathways and professional development that will encourage nurses to want to work as permanent staff on wards and to prevent drain to community teams (see training section). These developments should take into account any implications of the Agenda for Change programme.

❖ Trust HR departments should systematically gather information on why staff are leaving acute inpatient wards (exit interviews) with the aim of taking steps to improve retention.

❖ Trusts should prioritise recruitment and retention, analysing reasons for difficulties in recruitment and retention, and produce action plans specifically to address the identified difficulties.

❖ Workforce development confederations (WDCs) should support trusts on recruitment and retention initiatives, broader workforce development for inpatient staff and workforce planning for inpatient services to help them overcome the current difficulties.

Sickness, disciplinary action

❖ Trust HR departments should investigate the amount of disciplinary action occurring and its causes with a view to reducing this in the future where possible.

❖ Trust HR departments and line managers should review levels of sickness and absence and injuries resulting from violent incidents and identify what positive action can be taken to reduce sickness levels.

❖ Trusts should monitor the number of hours that permanent staff are working to ensure that individuals are not working excessive hours.

Ward housekeepers, administrative support

❖ RDCs should support trusts in looking at increased provision of ward housekeeping services as part of the New Ways of Working programme and share good practice examples across the regions.

❖ Trusts should review administrative support for wards as part of the review of staffing, particularly in those wards currently without any support.

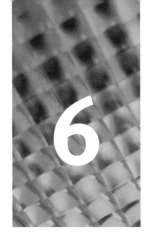

6 Impact of community teams on adult acute inpatient care

"It is now accepted that mental health services are most effective when delivery is within the context of the service user's local community. It is important that inpatient services maximise their connections to community services and vice versa."

Mental Health Policy Implementation Guide:
Adult Acute Inpatient Care Provision (DH, 2002a)

KEY FINDINGS

❖ 35% of ward managers reported that the client group on the ward had changed due to the development of community teams in the previous 12 months

❖ Of those that reported a change, 29% said that the client group was more severely ill

❖ 53% of ward managers reported that a crisis resolution team (CRT) admits to their ward

❖ 12% of ward managers who reported that CRTs admit to their ward stated that the CRT gatekeeps all admissions

❖ Only 38% of ward managers reported having good communication with community teams during the service user's admission

❖ 68% of ward managers fully understand the function and remits of community teams

CONTEXT

Much has been written in government policies and frameworks concerning the potential impact of community teams on the inpatient wards. The term community team covers a whole range of services including the well-established community mental health teams and the newer assertive outreach, crisis resolution and early intervention in psychosis teams. The *National Service Framework for Mental Health* (NSF-MH) says of assertive outreach teams that of "23 controlled studies, 61% reported significant reduction in hospital admissions" (DH, 1999a). One of the aims of early intervention in psychosis is to avoid hospitalisation (DH, 2001a) and the *NHS Plan* states that as a result of crisis resolution teams "pressure on acute inpatient units will be reduced by 30%" (DH, 2000a).

Although re-admissions occur for a variety of reasons, a high emergency re-admission rate may suggest that the level of mental health support provided in the community is inadequate. The development of new community teams, particularly crisis resolution teams, is likely to have an impact on relapse and re-admission rates. Admission and discharge data is collected locally within trusts and re-admission rates can be derived from this. This is one way in which the impact of community teams, particularly crisis resolution teams, can continue to be measured at a local or regional level.

In our survey we have not undertaken a full review of community teams. However, the survey does ask about the impact of teams on the inpatient ward, communication between the ward and community teams as well as the understanding of community function and remits. To put these findings in context we have included the dataset from Mental Health Service Mapping for Working Age Adults which we have analysed at both national and regional level.

Mental Health Service Mapping for Working Age Adults (Durham University) was established in 2000 and was developed to "contribute to monitoring the implementation of the mental health national service framework" (http://www dur.ac.uk/service.mapping/amh/index.php). Information about services is submitted twice a year to the service mapping by local implementation team (LIT) leads and provides amongst other information, the numbers of assertive outreach and crisis resolution teams. The following figures show data extrapolated from the mapping (as at April 2004).

Assertive outreach teams

In March 2003 there were 207 assertive outreach (AO) teams in place. The NHS Plan had a target of 220 assertive outreach teams to be in place by December 2003. By March 2004 there was actually a total of 259 assertive outreach teams in place. There had been a 27% national average increase in AO teams from March 2003 to March 2004. In terms of actual numbers, the highest number of teams were found in the South East and London which both had 43 teams as at March 2004. The lowest number of teams was to be found in the East Midlands, which had 18. However, it should be noted that there will be regional differences in the number of teams required due to varying local need and population size.

Figure 32 Comparison of assertive outreach teams March 2003/4 (from Durham Service Map)

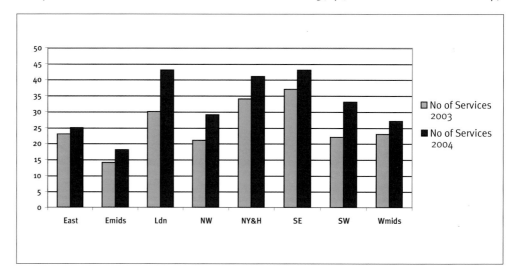

Crisis resolution teams   The NHS Plan stated that the target for crisis resolution teams was to have 335 in place by December 2004. In March 2004 the total of number teams in place was 170. The national average increase in CRTs from March 2003 to March 2004 had been 70%. In terms of actual numbers across the country, the highest number of CRTs was to be found in London, which had 31 teams by March 2004. Again, as with assertive outreach, the number of teams will relate to the local need of the region.

Figure 33   Comparison of crisis resolution teams March 2003/4 (from Durham Service Map)

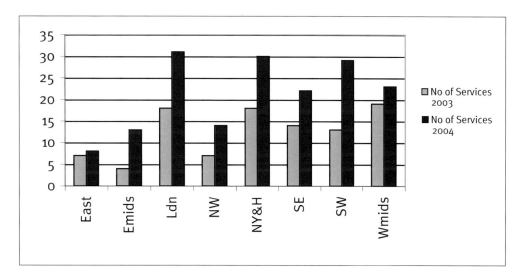

In March 2004, 72% of CRTs were providing a round-the-clock, 24/7 service, and in London and the West Midlands over 90% of CRTs were operating on a 24/7 basis.

Figure 34   Availability of crisis resolution teams at March 2004 (from Durham Service Map)

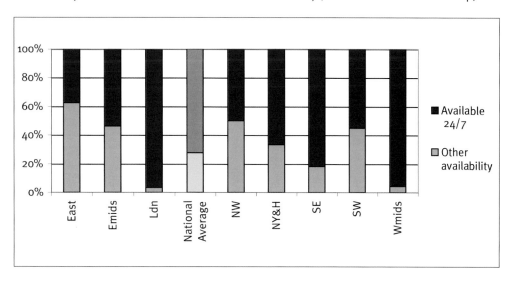

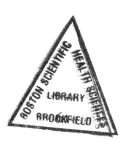

WHAT WE FOUND

The impact on
wards from 2003-4

Our results show that 53% of wards had a CRT admitting to their ward. Again, we analysed this by RDC to see if there were any significant regional differences. Those regions which had 50% or more wards with CRTs admitting to them were South West (75%), NY&H (66%), Eastern (60%) and West Midlands (51%). Although London had the highest percentage of CRTs, only 47% of ward managers reported that the teams were admitting to their wards.

Figure 35 Does a crisis resolution team admit to your ward? (310 responses)

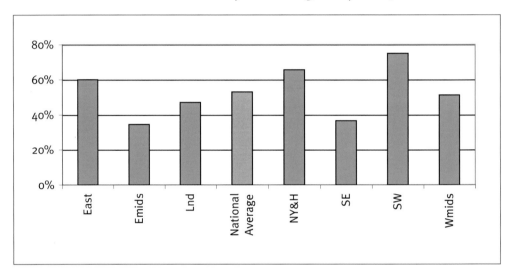

The MH-PIG identifies that the crisis resolution team should act as a 'gatekeeper' to mental health services (DH, 2001a). This means that service users should be seen by the CRT prior to admission to hospital. Although key targets for star ratings include fidelity to the model, gatekeeping is not one of the set criteria and therefore it is unclear how many CRTs are providing a full gatekeeping function (http://www. chi.nhs.uk/eng/ratings/2005/2005mentalhealth_KT.pdf). The specific importance of the gatekeeping function is highlighted by Niemiec and Tacchi who include this as one of the five essential criteria for providing positive impacts such as reduced bed occupancy, and decreases in admission and length of stay (Kennedy *et al.* 2003).

We found that 12% of ward managers who had CRTs admitting to the ward, reported that CRTs gatekept all admissions. Just over a quarter (26%) reported that the CRTs gatekept some of the admissions and 15% that CRTs gatekept most admissions. Looking at this by region, we see that London ward managers reported that 20% of the CRTs gatekept all admissions whereas in contrast only 4% of the East Midlands ward managers reported that CRTs gatekept all admissions. Nationally, 48% of ward managers stated that CRTs did not gatekeep admissions.

Figure 36 Does the crisis resolution team gatekeep admissions? (310 responses)

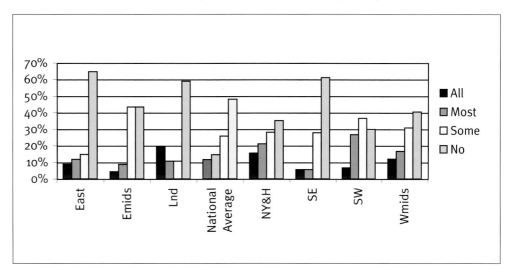

We then wanted to know how these ongoing changes in community teams had affected the wards on a national level over a 12-month period from 2003 to 2004. Perhaps surprisingly, 57% of ward managers did not perceive a change in the client group due to the development of community teams. This may be in part related to how closely the teams function to the model, such as their gatekeeping function. However, 35% thought that the client group had changed and the remainder reported being unsure about the impact.

To explore this further, we analysed this data at regional level and found that ward managers in the South West, London, NY&H and Eastern regions had noticed the most change in the client group. It is noteworthy that these regions had some of the highest percentage increases in CRTs and AO teams between March 2003 and 2004 and some of the highest percentages of ward managers stating that CRTs admit to their wards.

Figure 37 Has the client group changed due to developments in community services over the last 12 months? (307 responses)

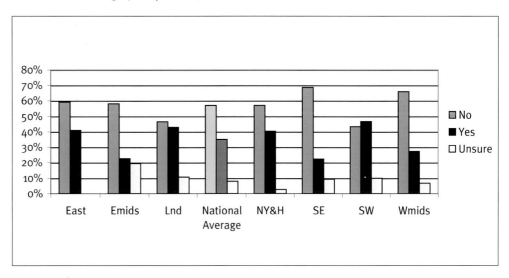

To understand this impact, we asked ward managers who had reported seeing a difference to categorise the way in which their client group had changed. We found that 29% reported that the service users on the ward were now more acutely ill and 22% reported seeing a difference in terms of the diagnoses of service users admitted. Smaller percentages reported a different age mix (4%) and a less acutely ill client group (3%).

These survey findings highlight the need for much more work to be undertaken to understand the impact of community teams on acute inpatient wards.

Communication between the ward and community teams

The aim of a whole systems approach is to provide ongoing seamless care that enables the smooth transition between teams in both the community and the ward. The key to any whole systems approach is clear and sustained communication between those teams. Establishing and maintaining good relationships and communication can be particularly difficult where there is high staff turnover and/or high numbers of agency and bank staff. However, many other factors may influence the level of communication. The MH-PIG Adult Acute states that "a positive policy on rotation of staff could help prevent/reduce barriers arising between services" and that "with the advent of new community acute treatment options there are local opportunities to improve service coherence and co-ordination by the creation of acute care nursing posts that work in both the inpatient and community treatment teams" (DH, 2002a).

The ward survey has enabled a baseline understanding of communication between the acute ward and community teams. Less than 10% of ward managers reported having excellent communication between their ward and community teams prior to and during admission and prior to discharge. An interesting trend seems to occur where community teams and wards are engaged with each other at the critical points of admission and discharge. We found that 50% of ward managers reported having good communication prior to discharge and 41% prior to admission. However engagement seems to drop off during an admission with only 38% reporting good communication during admission. This trend is further supported by *Acute Problems* which stated that "visits from community staff varied from 48 per cent of patients to an absolute low of none" (SCMH, 1998). Most worrying is the fact that a total of 16% of ward managers reported having either poor or very poor communication prior to admission with this rising to 19% during admission.

Figure 38 How good is communication between the ward and community teams? (310 responses)

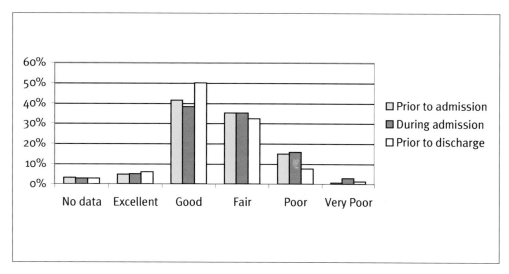

Crucial to the provision of seamless care by mental health services is the understanding of ward and team functions and remits. This self assessment of understanding by ward managers reveals that although 68% felt they fully understood the functions and remits of all community teams, 31% of ward managers only partially understood and 1% reported that they were not clear at all about the functions and remits of all teams.

Figure 39 How clear is your understanding of the functions and remits of all community teams? (310 responses)

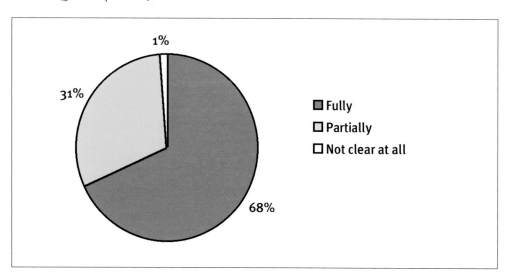

RECOMMENDATIONS

Whole systems approach
- ❖ Trusts should develop shared operational policies for acute inpatient and crisis resolution teams, highlighting the interdependent nature of these services, clarifying roles and functions, supporting effective communication and ensuring smooth transfer of information.

❖ Trusts should consider the suggestions in the Adult Acute MH-PIG (DH, 2002a) relating to single management of acute care services, staff rotation, acute care nursing posts that work in both inpatient and community treatment teams etc.

❖ Trusts should identify why and where there are breakdowns in communication between the wards and community teams e.g. during admission, and more specifically, with which teams and why.

❖ Trusts should provide information on the roles and functions of their teams, their likely impact and a 'service map' that demonstrates their interconnected nature to ensure that ward staff and community teams have a clear understanding of each other's remits.

Impact of community teams on acute inpatient wards

❖ Trusts should closely monitor the impact of community teams, especially crisis resolution teams, on acute wards. Most frequently measured are impact in terms of numbers of admissions, length of stay and bed occupancy. However, this study highlights that trusts should identify differences in severity of illness, diagnosis and age etc.

❖ Trusts should review staffing levels, skill mix and environmental needs in the light of the impact of the above.

❖ Trusts should provide adequate training and supervision to inpatient staff to ensure that they can meet the needs of a shifting client group.

Gatekeeping function

❖ Local implementation teams (LITs) should carefully consider the implications of crisis resolution teams not fulfilling a total gatekeeping function. As previously stated, this gatekeeping function is essential to reduce pressure on inpatient services.

❖ The Healthcare Commission should consider the evidence base for altering the current model of crisis resolution to include a specific criterion around the gatekeeping function.

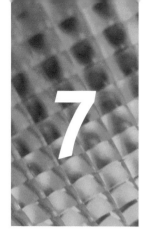

7 Training and development

"There is a need to recognise that undertaking this training is part of the job 'a real work factor'. Adequate training time must be planned and programmed in for all ward staff."

Mental Health Policy Implementation Guide:
Adult Acute Inpatient Care Provision (DH, 2002a)

KEY FINDINGS

❖ 77% of ward managers reported that their staff were given training on the 1983 Mental Health Act

❖ 93% of ward managers reported that staff were given training in risk asessment

❖ 89% of ward managers reported having a clear supervision and appraisal framework

❖ 75% of ward managers reported that all staff including unqualified staff have individual personal development plans

❖ 75% of ward managers reported that nursing staff were able to receive clinical supervision as often as needed

❖ The number of training days that each member of staff had completed in the previous 12 months was highly variable

❖ Less than half of ward managers reported that there was a career development programme for all staff within inpatient services

CONTEXT

The introduction to *Working Together, Learning Together: A Framework for Lifelong Learning for the NHS* states that "Lifelong Learning and development are key to delivering the Government's vision of patient centred care in the NHS" (DH, 2001b). Lifelong learning is not just about training but also includes continuing personal development (CPD). The Commission for Health Improvement (CHI) reported that it found a strong commitment by trusts to staff development (Healthcare Commission, 2003). However, it acknowledged that there were difficulties in releasing staff for training due to service pressures.

In June 2004, *Acute Inpatient Mental Health Care: Education, Training & Continuing Professional Development for All* was published by NIMHE. This publication is a supplement to the *Mental Health Policy Implementation Guide: Adult Acute*

Inpatient Care Provision (MH-PIG Adult Acute) and acknowledges the lack of training programmes specifically aimed at acute inpatient care (DH, 2002a). The training guidance aims "to make current training and development opportunities more relevant and available to inpatient practitioners" (Clarke, 2004).

Our survey takes a look at just some aspects of the training of acute inpatient staff but does not explore the quality of training currently provided. Our service user feedback on the survey findings echoes one of a number of recommendations in the training guidance that "service users and carers must be involved in the design, delivery and evaluation of training and education programmes for acute inpatient care" (Clarke, 2004).

WHAT WE FOUND

Almost 100% of ward managers across the regions reported that there was evidence of participation in continued professional training and development on the ward. We asked about some specifics of the training as follows:

The Mental Health Act

The majority of ward managers (77%) confirmed that nursing staff did receive training in the 1983 Mental Health Act and the revised code of practice. In NY&H region, this was confirmed by all of the ward managers who took part in the survey. Where Mental Health Act training was given 67% of ward managers confirmed that this was repeated on an annual basis. It should also be recognised that the impending Mental Health Bill will have significant training implications for all acute staff.

Training in information collection and analysis

With NHS organisations now expected to monitor and improve the quality of care given, it is likely that ward staff will be increasingly involved in audit and research. Training specifically in information collection and analysis with regards to audit and research is currently being given to staff on between 21% and 40% of wards across the regions.

Training relating to safety issues

We found that 93% of ward managers reported that staff were given training in risk assessment. Across the regions this ranged from 90% of ward managers in NY&H region to 98% of ward managers in London.

We then asked about training in the management of imminent and actual violence and found that 95% of ward managers reported that staff were given this training. Across the regions this ranged from 89% of ward managers in the South West to 98% of ward managers in the West Midlands.

Third, we asked about training in breakaway techniques and/or restraint measures. We found that 98% of ward managers confirmed that staff were given this training. Across the regions this ranged from 96% of ward managers in NY&H region to 100% of ward managers in the Eastern, East Midlands, South West and West Midlands regions.

Our survey does not show whether all staff are being given the safety training or whether the training was only offered to a few staff. It also does not show how frequently training is updated.

The quality of training is vital. To ensure that training in the recognition, prevention and management of aggression and violence is consistently of high standard, NIMHE is developing proposals for a "national accreditation and regulation scheme for both trainers and education and training programmes" (NIMHE, 2004).

Number of training days

We asked about the average number of training days that staff had completed over the previous 12 months (2003 to 2004) and we found considerable variation both within and across the regions. Ward managers reported the average number of training days as follows:

❖ 41% reported the average as more than 5 days

❖ 35% reported the average as 4-5 days

❖ 24% reported the average as 1-3 days

The South East and South West reported the lowest average numbers of training days taken over the 12 months, with ward managers stating that the largest proportion of staff had received between 1 and 3 days training. Where there were low numbers of training days such as 1-3 days, it may suggest that some staff were receiving only essential training such as in control and restraint and/or the Mental Health Act. It should be noted that this survey does not ask about the types of training nor their quality.

Figure 40 On average how many training days has each member of staff completed over the past 12 months? (310 responses)

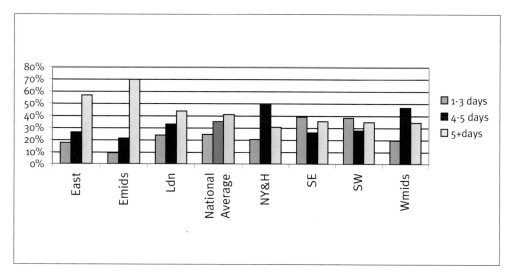

We found that 96% of ward managers reported that the ward had links with higher education centres and trust training and development centres. This is an encouraging finding particularly if these links are well established with education centres taking an active role in informing and facilitating training for ward staff.

Teaching sessions for students

Nationally, 76% of wards were able to provide regular teaching sessions for students. Provision of teaching sessions may help to make the acute inpatient ward learning experience a positive one and therefore play an important part in the future recruitment of student nurses onto acute wards when they qualify. In our survey, 73 wards throughout the country were unable to provide these teaching sessions. This could be for a number of reasons including staff shortages which make it difficult to ensure adequate staff cover for the ward whilst releasing staff for training. This cycle of recruitment and retention difficulties will be repeated if wards are unable to retain the students that they train.

Supervision, appraisals, personal development planning and career development

One of the goals of *Working Together, Learning Together* is that employers have "coherent appraisal systems and extension of personal development plans to all staff" (DH, 2001b) and the MH-PIG Adult Acute states that "effective staff support and supervision arrangements must be in place" (DH, 2002a). The issue of supervision training for those giving supervision is identified in both the NW Acute Ward Survey (Ryan, 2003) and in the London HAS report (2003).

We asked ward managers if there was a clear supervision and appraisal framework and 89% confirmed that there was. In the Eastern region, all of the ward managers who took part in the survey confirmed that this was in place.

We found that three quarters of ward managers reported that there was adequate supervision for nursing staff. The London HAS report (2003) points out the difficulties for staff supervision if there is insufficient staff cover, stating that "while there is a possibility during shift crossover times, these spaces tend to be occupied with other activities, including handover, business and management meeting and the volume of supervision required could not be accommodated in these times".

Figure 41 Are nursing staff currently able to receive clinical supervision as often as they need? (228 responses)

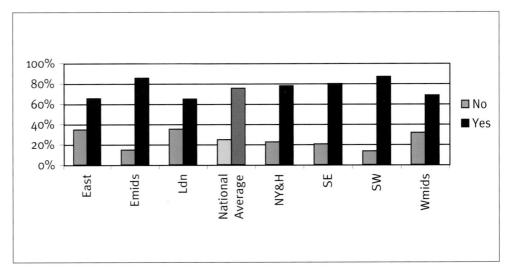

We asked whether all staff (including unqualified) had individual personal development plans (PDPs) and nationally 75% of ward managers confirmed that they did. Survey responses from Eastern region show a lower than average positive response at 45%. This is particularly interesting given the region's exceptionally high positive response on supervision and appraisal.

Figure 42   Do all staff (inc. unqualified) have individual personal development plans? (310 responses)

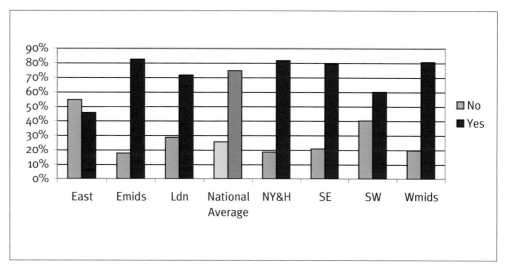

The MH-PIG Adult Acute states that "attention needs to be given to improved career structure and incentives across the full complement of inpatient nursing grades" (DH, 2002a). We asked ward managers whether a clear career development programme was offered to staff within inpatient services. The regional responses show some differences and London (at 59%) has a higher than average 'yes' response. However, in all other regions, fewer than 50% of ward managers responded that they did have a clear career development programme for all staff in inpatient services. This has serious implications for both the recruitment and retention of nurses and other workers in the acute inpatient setting and needs to be reviewed alongside practices relating to supervision, appraisal and personal development planning.

Figure 43   Is there a clear career development programme offered to staff within inpatient services? (310 responses)

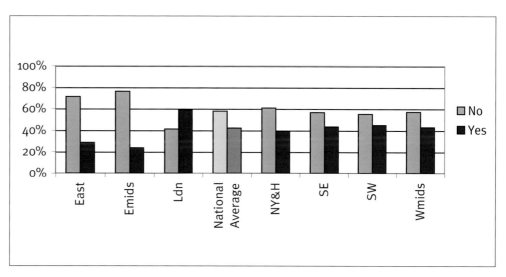

RECOMMENDATIONS

Training – overview

❖ Acute care forums (ACFs)/education providers/ward managers with trust support should design and develop training and educational programmes based on the core capabilities of acute inpatient care (Clarke, 2004).

❖ RDCs/ACFs/training and education providers should explore the current training provided to staff with regard to appropriateness and quality, using the Northern Centre *National Continuous Quality Improvement Tool for Mental Health Education* (2003) available as a pdf on the North East, Yorkshire & Humber development centre website. (http://www.nimheneyh.org.uk/subject.cfm?secid=27&subid=108).

❖ ACFs/trusts should look at the number of training days taken on acute inpatient wards as well as which staff are provided with training opportunities. This review should look also at reasons why low numbers of training days are taken and any action required. Training needs to be taken into account when looking at staffing levels.

❖ SHA education leads/trusts/nurse education providers/modern matrons/ward managers should review the provision of regular teaching sessions for students and help facilitate regular teaching sessions where they do not currently occur.

❖ Trusts should consider the use of systematic whole ward, multidisciplinary training.

Training – safety

❖ Trusts should look at the safety training provided to ward staff. Training should be provided for all ward staff, kept regularly updated and be of high quality.

Training – Mental Health Act

❖ Trusts should ensure that all staff are provided with regular training in the Mental Health Act. When a revised Mental Health Bill is finalised then all staff must be updated.

Appraisals and personal development planning

❖ Trusts/ACFs/human resources departments/ward managers should ensure that regular supervision is provided alongside appraisals and personal development planning for all staff. Where this is not currently occurring they should find out why and help to facilitate change in practice.

❖ Trusts/human resource departments should review how clear career development programmes can be implemented and their implications for recruitment and retention on acute inpatient wards. Examples of good practice should be shared across regions and release of staff for specific acute inpatient training and education should be explored.

For further recommendations please refer to the publication: *Acute Inpatient Mental Health Care: Education, Training & Continuing Professional Development for All* (Clarke, 2004) published by NIMHE.

8 Information technology

KEY FINDINGS

❖ 81% of ward managers reported that all of the ward team had computer access

❖ Internet and email access was restricted on some wards to certain staff

❖ 97% of ward managers reported that some or all of the staff had received training in computers and available programs

❖ 25% of ward staff routinely accessed the electronic care programme approach system (e-CPA), but agency and bank staff often did not have access

---

CONTEXT

Information technology is fast becoming integral in the running of the acute inpatient ward. The Government is making a huge investment in technology for the NHS with its ambitious National Programme for Information Technology (NPfIT). This aims to "make a significant difference to improving the patient experience and the delivery of care and services" (http://www.publications.doh.gov.uk/ipu/programme/index.htm) and one of the key deliverables is electronic care records for service users. The Department of Health publication *Delivering 21st Century IT Support for the NHS: National Strategic Programme* (2002c) details the proposed modernisation of IT and how it will help with delivery of the *NHS Plan*. In our survey, we wanted to find about the current use of technology on acute inpatient wards.

WHAT WE FOUND

The ward team included all staff groups and in our survey most ward managers (81%) reported having computer access for everyone on the ward. On the remaining wards access was available to some staff. Our survey did not identify which staff did not have access and this may vary across regions. No wards were reported to be without a computer.

Nationally, 67% of ward managers reported that everyone on the ward had access to the internet and 31% that wards had internet access for only some staff. Five ward managers, in Eastern, NY&H, South East and West Midlands regions, reported having no internet access on the ward. Lack of internet access limits the ward staff's ability to gain access to external sources of information such as the websites of the Department of Health, NIMHE and other mental health and professional organisations, all of which could potentially be valuable sources of research, information and networks for acute inpatient staff.

Figure 44   How many team members have access to the internet on the ward? (309 responses)

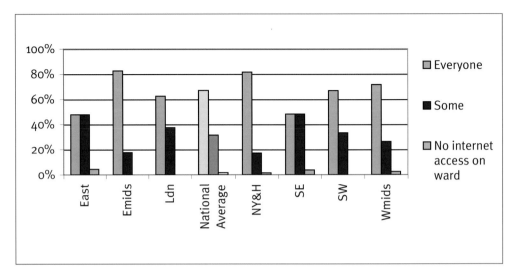

A similar picture is presented with regard to internal email access for staff on the wards. 63% of ward managers reported that everyone had access to the internal email system and 36% reported that only some staff had access. There were four wards where managers reported they did not have an internal email system. Many trusts provide a range of information via internal email and staff members frequently use email to communicate with colleagues. Anecdotal evidence shows that emails may be sent to colleagues within a trust with the erroneous assumption that the intended recipient has access to email. Limited access has implications for both information dissemination and service delivery.

Figure 45   Do all team members have access to the internal email on the ward? (308 responses)

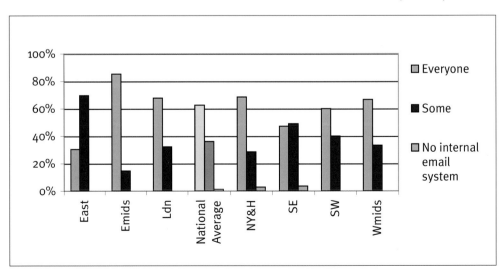

We then asked about training in the use of the computer and software packages and found that 16% of ward managers stated that everyone in the ward team had received training. 81% of ward managers reported that some staff had received training. Nationally, nine ward managers reported that none of the team had received computer training and these were found across all regions except West Midlands.

There may be a number of reasons why not all staff received training, such as: being new in post, difficulty in releasing staff from the ward, reluctance to undertake training, or a limited number of trainers to cover the trust etc.

Figure 46 How many of the team on the ward have had training in the use of the computer and software? (308 responses)

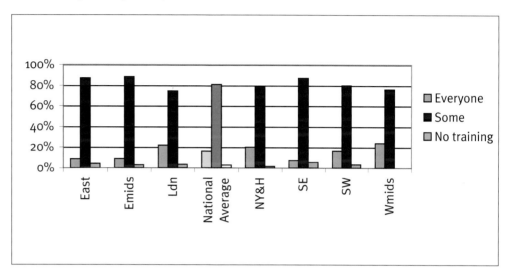

Trusts' care programme approach (CPA) systems implementation is measured by the Healthcare Commission and informs calculations for star ratings. The Healthcare Commission specifically asks about electronic CPA. Nationally, 25% of ward managers reported that staff routinely accessed e-CPA. In the East Midlands, it is noteworthy that a total of 56% (15 ward managers) reported that staff routinely accessed e-CPA and this higher percentage is echoed in the high average percentage of computer access and training in the region.

Figure 47 Do staff routinely access e-CPA? (298 responses)

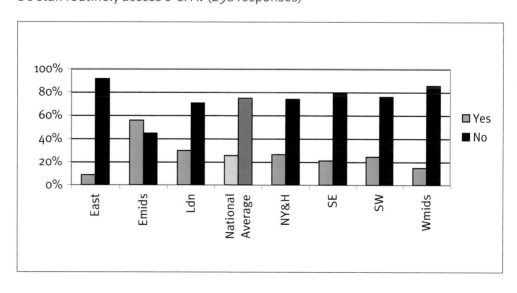

On wards where staff were accessing e-CPA, we wanted to find out whether this included bank and agency staff, and the vast majority reported that it did not. Of the 73 wards where staff used e-CPA, bank and agency staff had access to it in just 11. There may be a number of reasons why bank and agency staff did not access e-CPA such as a lack of password access to computers and/or a lack of training on how to use the computer system. As trusts continue to develop e-CPA, it does raise questions about how this can be fully and effectively implemented given the high number of bank and agency staff that are frequently required in mental health trusts throughout the country. Where bank and agency staff do not access e-CPA, it raises further concerns about how they input and retrieve information relating to the service users for whom they are caring.

RECOMMENDATIONS

IT policies and ward staff involvement

❖ Trusts should review policies on internet and internal email access for all staff groups. Where internal email is not made available to all staff then formal systems need to be in place to ensure that information is provided to those without access.

❖ Trusts should ensure that ward managers/ward staff are involved in the development of IT policies and in the creation of IT documentation, particularly documentation to be used by the ward.

IT training

❖ Trusts/acute care forums (ACFs)/ward managers should review staff computer training and ensure that all staff complete computer training. This is particularly important as trusts move towards electronic records.

Bank and agency staff

❖ Where e-CPA is implemented, trusts/ACFs should explore whether bank and agency staff can access the e-CPA and address their training needs. Where bank and agency staff do not currently have access then trusts/ACFs should investigate what this means for both care and administrative processes.

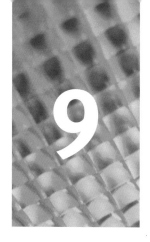

9 Policies

"It is essential that there are shared values, principles and processes across the whole service system. There needs to be a clear set of locally negotiated and agreed operational policies covering specifically the entirety of acute care as it stands at present and that will lead on to incorporating the new elements of service as they come into being."

Mental Health Policy Implementation Guide:
Adult Acute Inpatient Care Provision (DH, 2002a)

KEY FINDINGS

❖ Nationally, the majority of wards reported that they had the policies listed in our survey questionnaire and staff had been made aware of them

❖ 100% of wards had policies of which staff had been made aware, for disciplinaries and grievances, and for complaints

❖ A small percentage of ward managers across the country were unsure whether they had some of the listed policies

CONTEXT

National and local policies are made to affect and guide action, to provide structure for practice, to drive and instigate change and to set standards. We wanted to gain an understanding of the policies in place on wards. We provided a list of policies in the survey questionnaire and asked wards to say 'yes', 'no' or 'unsure' to indicate whether they had these policies on their ward.

There is likely to be a small amount of variation across the country, as certain policies will be driven by local needs. National and local policy recommendations are found in the *Mental Health Policy Implementation Guide: Adult Acute Inpatient Care Provision* (MH-PIG Adult Acute) and a range of other guidance (DH, 2002a). It is not the remit of this report to specify all the policies that should be in place and our list is not definitive. Our aim is to highlight areas relating to policy which may require review by regions and trusts.

WHAT WE FOUND

Nationally, we found that the vast majority of wards had our listed policies in place and that staff had been aware of them. There were two policies that 100% (302 responses) of wards had in place:

1. disciplinaries and grievances

2. complaints

Although the majority of ward managers reported that they had the policies listed below, there were small percentages across the regions that either did not have or were unsure whether they had them:

- ❖ Bullying and harassment

- ❖ Equal opportunities

- ❖ Privacy and dignity

- ❖ Management of medical emergencies

- ❖ Management of psychiatric emergencies

- ❖ Management of accidents/incidents

- ❖ Clinical and management review after emergencies

- ❖ Searches of users and their property

- ❖ Visitors to the ward

- ❖ Children visiting the ward

- ❖ Promotion of safety on the ward

- ❖ Observation of people who are assessed as being at high risk of threatening or harmful behaviour

- ❖ Prevention of violence on the ward

- ❖ Management of violent incidents on the ward

- ❖ Safety of women on the ward

- ❖ Use of and recording the use of restraints on the ward

- ❖ Use and recording of seclusion

- ❖ Policy for service users who go absent without leave from the ward

It is very encouraging that so many wards have policies in place and that staff have been made aware of them, but it is of concern that there are a small number of trusts/wards that are not following mental health policy implementation guidance and/or wards where there is uncertainty about policies. Those wards where there is uncertainty about having policies may still be following positive practice/trust guidelines. However, given high staff turnover and agency usage on many wards, clarity about existing policies and ensuring policy information is kept up-to-date would seem advisable if not essential.

RECOMMENDATIONS

Updating and disseminating policies

❖ Trusts/acute care forums (ACFs) should ensure that all policies are kept updated, ensuring that all local managers and ward staff are kept informed.

❖ Trusts should ensure that staff are exposed to trust policies as part of the induction process.

❖ Trusts/ward managers/practice development leads should ensure that where policies are only available via the intranet, all grades of staff and agency/bank staff are able to access the policies. Hard copies should be available as necessary.

❖ RDCs/ACFs should facilitate the sharing of policies and protocols across the regions.

Implementation

❖ Trusts/ACFs should consider a systematic auditing of trust policy awareness and implementation which incorporates service user participation and service user-led audit.

❖ Trusts/ACFs should ensure that ward staff are aware of the implications of not having access to and/or implementing policies.

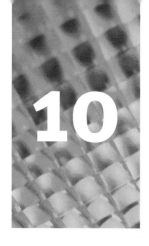

10 Safety issues

"Operational policies ... must be clear and consistent about process and responsibilities regarding:

❖ Creating and maintaining a safe environment for users, visitors and staff."

Mental Health Policy Implementation Guide:
Adult Acute Inpatient Care Provision (DH, 2002a)

KEY FINDINGS

❖ 86% of ward managers considered their ward to be a safe place

❖ 82% of ward managers reported that their wards could be locked and 84% of those reported that this facility was used

❖ 81% of ward managers reported there was a policy for locking the ward

❖ 28% of ward managers reported that seclusion was used on the ward

❖ 72% of ward managers reported that there was a policy for the use and recording of seclusion

❖ 82% of ward managers reported having access to a psychiatric intensive care unit (PICU)

❖ Many wards struggled to provide data on incidents relating to violence, suicide, absconsions, deliberate acts of self-harm and homicide

CONTEXT

There is much recent evidence to suggest that problems associated with violence in mental health inpatient services are widespread. Mind's *Ward Watch* campaign report published in 2004 states that 27% of respondents to their survey felt unsafe in hospital. They found that "51 percent of recent or current inpatients reported being verbally or physically threatened during their stay".

Early findings from the Royal College of Psychiatrists' Research Unit's 2003-5 Healthcare Commission-funded programme *The National Audit of Violence: towards safer and more therapeutic residential care for people with mental health problems or learning disability* indicate that many service users, staff, and visitors are being exposed to highly unsafe situations that are outside of their control (Royal College of Psychiatrists, unpublished).

The National Patient Safety Agency's (NPSA) National Reporting and Learning System (NRLS) showed a "high number of mental health patient safety incidents related to inpatient wards" and in August 2004 the NPSA announced that they will be undertaking a project to "improve the safety of mental health service users by creating a safer environment on acute psychiatric wards" (http://www.npsa.nhs.uk).

In relation to the reporting of incidents, Mind (2004) found that only 37% of those "threatened, or who had been the victim of verbal abuse, violence, racism or sexual harassment while in hospital, reported this incident to a staff member". In its round of inspection visits, CHI found that "trusts generally have good systems for incident reporting and reviewing serious untoward incidents, including suicides, but that there was little evidence of feedback to staff, dissemination of learning or trend analysis" (Healthcare Commission, 2003). They also found that there were different approaches to the prevention and management of violence and aggression whereby in some areas "staff accept violent behaviour as the norm, on others zero tolerance approaches are used" (Healthcare Commission, 2003).

In response to concerns, NIMHE has published the *Mental Health Policy Implementation Guide: Developing Positive Practice to Support the Safe and Therapeutic Management of Aggression and Violence in Mental Health In-patient Settings* (2004) and this includes positive practice standards. NIMHE will be writing definitive guidance now the National Institute for Clinical Excellence (NICE) have published guidelines on *Violence: The short-term management of disturbed/ violent behaviour in in-patient psychiatric settings and emergency departments* (2005).

In our *Acute Care 2004* survey, we wanted to gain some baseline information about safety issues and reporting of incidents on the wards. The difficulties that ward managers had in responding to these questions can be seen in the slightly lower response rates for this section.

WHAT WE FOUND

In the NW Acute Ward survey, it was found that 73% of ward managers thought the ward safe (Ryan, 2003). We wanted to find out from our survey whether ward managers thought that their ward was a safe place for both service users and staff. Responses were on the whole positive with 86% of ward managers stating that they considered their ward to be safe. Responses by region ranged from 72% in the East Midlands to 95% in the West Midlands. The results from our survey are in sharp contrast to recent service user surveys carried out by Mind (2004) and the National Patient Safety Agency (http://www.npsa.nhs.uk), which found that service users did not feel safe on acute inpatient wards. Given this difference in perception, it is strongly recommended that additional work is carried out at a regional/local level to obtain service user views.

Figure 48   In general do you consider the ward to be a safe place for patients and staff? (302 responses)

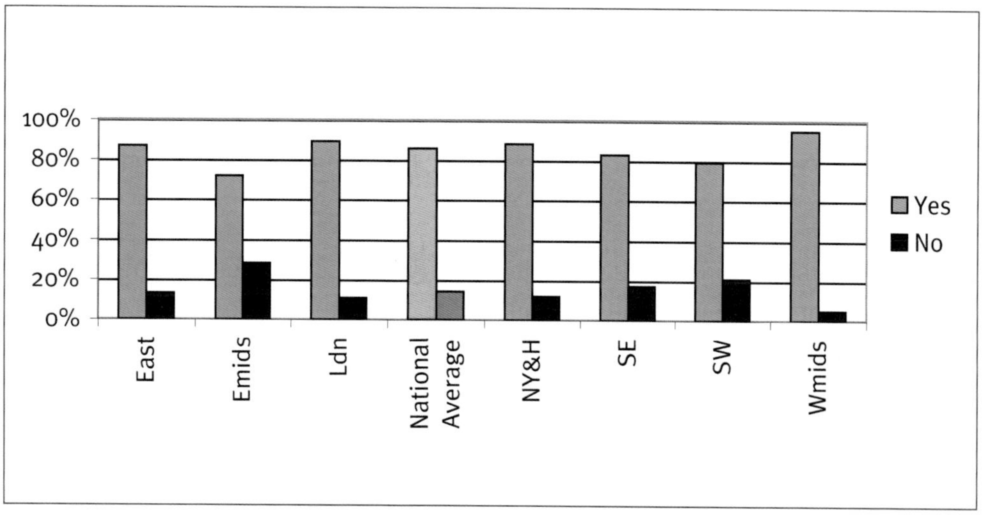

Locking the ward   Locking acute inpatient wards means that service users who are not detained under a Mental Health Act section and visitors to the ward will need to find a member of staff to open the door for them. Bowers (2003) suggests in his article *Runaway patients* that "many wards have now become permanently locked in order to prevent absconding" but that this is "a new phenomenon in the UK ... not supported by the current Mental Health Act Code of Conduct". The London HAS report (2003) found that "increased security also tended to follow from some form of incident such as an attack on service users or staff from a person not associated with the hospital. Locking the ward can therefore be about protection of those inside the ward and/or about keeping service users in".

We wanted to find out firstly whether the ward could be locked and 82% of ward managers confirmed that it could. The percentage of wards that could be locked was highest in London at 95%.

Figure 49   Is the ward lockable? (305 responses)

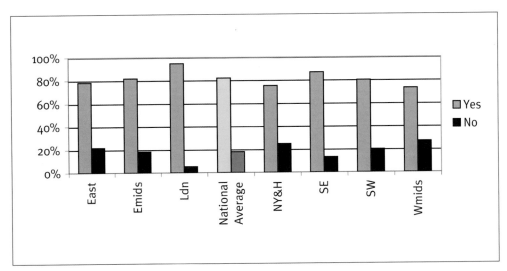

We then asked if this facility was used and 84% of ward managers confirmed that it was. There were small regional percentage differences with use of this facility but overall in most places where there was the facility to lock the ward it was used.

Figure 50   If the ward is lockable is this facility used? (241 responses)

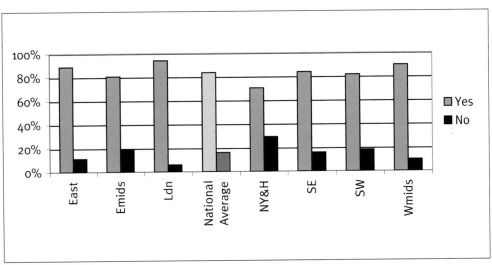

We wanted to see how frequently the ward was locked. It occurred frequently on 37% of wards, occasionally on 30% of wards and rarely on 33%. Looking at the average percentage usage, London region wards were locked most frequently and those in the South West least.

Figure 51   If the ward is locked how frequently does this happen? (190 responses)

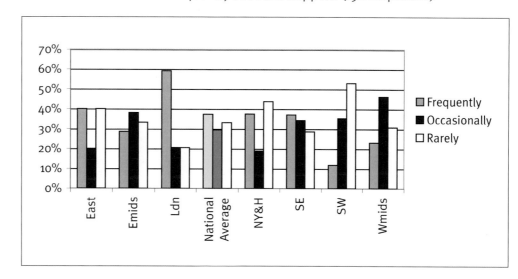

We wanted to know if there was a policy for locking the ward and 81% of ward managers responded that there was.

Figure 52   Is there a policy for locking the ward? (289 responses)

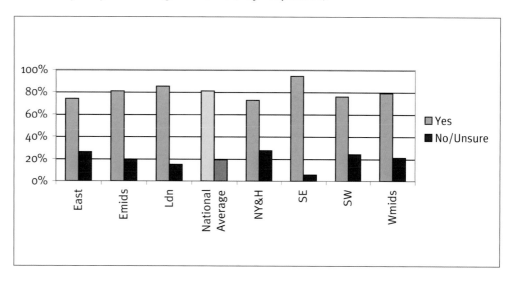

Nationally 9% of ward managers reported that the wards were locked but they did not have or were unsure if there was a policy for locking the ward. Where wards do not have a policy, this leaves them vulnerable to criticism.

Use of seclusion   Seclusion involves locking a service user into a room when they become aggressive or violent and we wanted to find out how widely this practice was used. In total 28% of ward managers reported that seclusion was used on the ward. The highest percentage was in the East Midlands at 48%.

85

Figure 53   Is seclusion used on the ward? (304 responses)

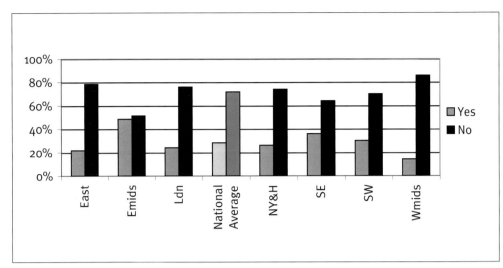

We also asked all ward managers if they had a policy on the use and recording of seclusion. We found that nearly a quarter of ward managers were either without a policy or unsure if they had one. Nationally, there were three wards which reported using seclusion but were without/unsure if they had a policy.

Figure 54   Is there a policy on the use and recording of seclusion? (308 responses)

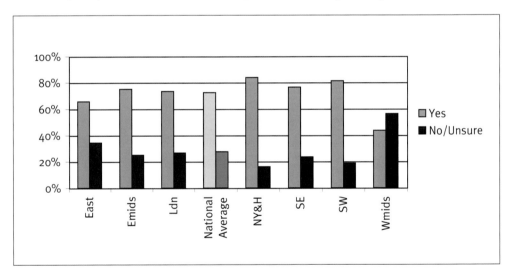

Use of psychiatric intensive care units (PICUs)

"Psychiatric intensive care is for patients compulsorily detained usually in secure conditions, who are in an acutely disturbed phase of a serious mental disorder. There is an associated loss of capacity for self-control, with a corresponding increase in risk, which does not enable their safe, therapeutic management and treatment in a general open acute ward" (DH, 2002d). The *Mental Health Policy Implementation Guide: Adult Acute Inpatient Care Provision* (MH-PIG Adult Acute) states that "every acute inpatient facility should have access to an identified PICU in their area" (DH, 2002a).

We found that 82% of ward managers stated that they had access to a PICU or an intensive care area. This still leaves 18% without access.

Figure 55   Does your ward have access to a PICU or an intensive care area? (291 responses)

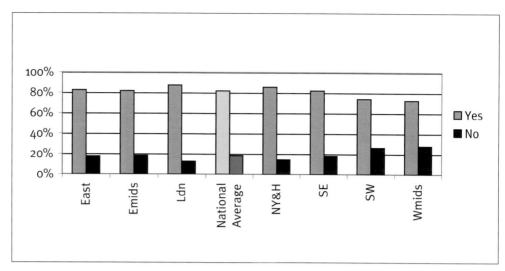

We wanted to gain some idea of how often ward managers had to find a bed in a PICU for patients on the ward in the previous 12 months. We found that 22% had frequently had to do this, 52% occasionally, 20% rarely and 6% never. What we do not know is whether provision of PICU beds matched service user need.

Figure 56   How often have you had to place patients in a PICU in the past 12 months? (231 responses)

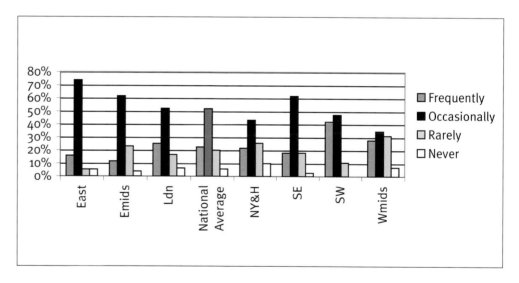

Critical incident review and incident recording   In our survey we asked ward managers whether critical incident debriefing was used on the ward. However, the new NICE guidelines on *Disturbed/ Violent Behaviour* which cover "Incident Reporting and Post-Incident Reviews following Rapid Tranquillisation, Physical Interventions and Seclusion" have since been published. The new guidelines recommend that one-off critical incident debriefing should not be used, but a post-incident review process should be undertaken instead, and for this reason we are not including the results of the question on critical incident debriefing. The guidelines state that a review should take place as soon after the incident as possible and at least within 72 hours, and involve appropriately skilled staff. The aim of the review is to be a learning process which enables feelings about the incident to be listened to, support provided for those involved, and a review of what lessons can be learned (NICE, 2005).

We wanted to find out about the numbers of recorded incidents in the previous 12 months relating to violence, suicide, acts of deliberate self-harm, absconding and homicide, split by gender. In the Eastern and East Midlands regions the majority of ward managers could provide data but this was not the case for all other regions. For example, the national average percentage of ward managers who were unable/ did not provide data on violent incidents is 61% and there are similar patterns of low responses for all types of incidents. With such low responses to this part of the survey we have not included the findings. Some feedback from ward managers on this was that there was a lack of or difficulty in obtaining feedback on incident reporting rather than a lack of actual incident recording. This would suggest that trust clinical governance and audit processes with regard to incident recording may not be informing service delivery and that data on incidents is not readily available to ward managers. This type of information is essential in the pursuit of preventing violence. The Counter Fraud and Security Management Services and NPSA are currently both engaged in developing systems of reporting.

Figure 57 Wards provision of data on number of violent incidents in past 12 months (310 responses)

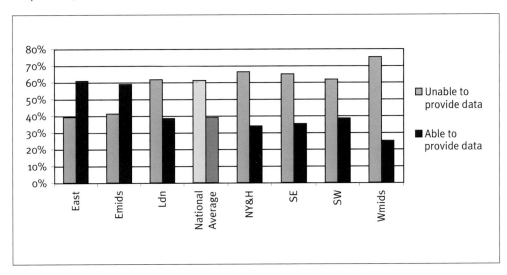

RECOMMENDATIONS

Reviewing safety ❖ Trusts should undertake anonymised surveys to find out how safe staff, service users and visitors feel the wards to be and why. This information should be used to understand problems, to identify positive practice and to assist in the creation of safer and more therapeutic environments as appropriate. The *National Audit of Violence* audit tools are available on the Royal College of Psychiatrists website at http://www.rcpsych.ac.uk/cru/audithm.htm

❖ Strategic health authorities/NIMHE/RDCs should encourage acute care forums (ACFs) to undertake audit and surveys to explore why wards are being locked.

This needs to include finding out why some wards do not have or do not use this facility and must also include input from service users and carers.

❖ NIMHE should ensure that the frequent locking of doors is made known to those involved in the development of the new code of practice.

Policies   ❖ Trusts should develop policies, where they do not exist, on the use of seclusion and locking of wards in consultation with service users and ward staff.

❖ Trusts should ensure that the new *Mental Health Policy Implementation Guide: Developing Positive Practice to Support the Safe and Therapeutic Management of Aggression and Violence in Mental Health In-patient Settings* (NIMHE, 2004) informs practice and that the new NICE guidelines (2005) on *Disturbed/Violent Behaviour* are implemented.

PICU   ❖ SHAs/PCTs/trusts should look at the provision of PICU beds and the impact of provision or the lack of provision on acute inpatient wards.

Clinical governance   ❖ Trust clinical governance leads should ensure that all incidents involving staff and/or service users are accurately recorded and that there is a process of feedback and review at trust management *and* ward level.

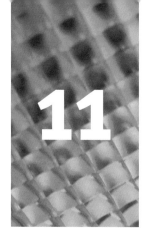

11 Care Programme Approach

"Effective care planning provides an ongoing framework for properly assessed and co-ordinated care and risk management; service user and carer involvement and communication amongst disciplines and across care settings."

Mental Health Policy Implementation Guide:
Adult Acute Inpatient Care Provision (DH, 2002a)

KEY FINDINGS

❖ The majority of ward managers reported that the assessment process included a range of key information not just related to mental health

❖ 60% of ward managers reported that they had access to crisis plans developed in the community

❖ 59% of ward managers reported that they did not have access to advance directives drawn up by the service user

❖ 87% of ward managers confirmed that CMHTs and GPs were notified of admissions and discharges within 72 hours

❖ 55% of ward managers said service users always had a written treatment plan produced within 72 hours

❖ 99% of ward managers stated that service users could invite an advocate, carer and/or family members to care plan discussions, and that they were made aware of this

CONTEXT

The Care Programme Approach (CPA) was introduced in 1990 as the framework for the care of people with mental health needs. It was revised and integrated with local authority Care Management in 1999 to form a single care co-ordination approach for adults of working age with mental health needs, to be used as the format for assessment, care planning and review of care by health and social care staff in all settings, including inpatient care. The Department of Health policy booklet also outlines its criteria for establishing a 'robust CPA', identifying standards which trusts must implement (DH, 1999c).

The Care Programme Approach Association (CPAA) was established in 1996 to support the implementation, operation and development of the CPA. They have published national standards, and a tool for auditing the CPA which provides information on service users' and carers' experiences of the CPA, as well as assessing the quality of the documentation and providing guidance for CPA care co-ordinators (http://www.cpaa.co.uk). The Department of Health also has *An Audit Pack for Monitoring the Care Programme Approach* (available from http://www. publications.doh.gov.uk/mentalhealth/auditpack.pdf).

There are two levels of CPA, standard and enhanced. The standard CPA is for people who need only low-level support, usually from just one agency. It is also for people who pose no risk to themselves or others. Those on enhanced CPA have more complex needs, usually require input from more than one agency such as health and housing, and are more likely to disengage with services. People on enhanced CPA are more likely to have severe mental health problems, and to be at risk of harming themselves or others.

We wanted to find out some basic information from ward managers regarding use of the CPA. Although having a CPA Care Plan is not a guarantee that users' needs have been adequately assessed or that planned interventions will be implemented effectively, it is generally regarded as a reasonable proxy measure for good practice. This survey does not aim to assess the quality of the CPA and related documentation. The Healthcare Commission is responsible for assessing trusts' performance on CPA systems implementation (i.e. that care plans are held on a central database which is regularly updated and available 24 hours a day) and on the CPA/complex care indicator (i.e. the CPA status of service users receiving complex specialist mental health care).

WHAT WE FOUND

CPA We asked if the wards had a standard policy for CPA that included a standard/enhanced approach and 97% (294 responses) of ward managers confirmed they had. This was 100% for both Eastern and South East regions.

We wanted to find out if there was an identified lead person responsible for implementing and monitoring CPA. The lead is responsible for reporting to the trust board on local implementation of the CPA. Often this is an administrative post within the trust and sometimes the role is combined with that of the Mental Health Act Manager. We found that 83% (303 responses) of ward managers confirmed that there was an identified lead person and in the East Midlands this was confirmed by 100% of ward managers.

Assessment We wanted to know whether the assessment process included a range of key information. Standard Four of the *National Service Framework for Mental Health* (NSF-MH) states that assessment should cover "psychiatric, psychological and social functioning, risk to the individual and others, including previous violence and criminal record, any needs from co-morbidity, and personal circumstances including family or other carers, housing, financial and occupational status" (DH, 1999a).

Table 6   What does assessment take into account?

Does assessment take into account:	Yes
Cultural preferences	98%
Diagnosis	96%
Forensic history	98%
Language	99%
Physical illness	95%
Physical impairment/disability	96%
Previous assessment	96%
Risk assessment	100%
Sensory impairment/disability	92%

These findings are on the whole very positive but it is of concern that the assessment process did not include all the above areas in 100% of cases. The need to assess physical health needs is well documented and the NSF-MH cites the National Psychiatric Morbidity Survey which showed "high levels of physical ill health and higher rates of death amongst those with mental health problems compared to the rest of the population" (DH, 1999a). Shift is a 5-year initiative being run by NIMHE to "tackle stigma and discrimination surrounding mental health issues" and one area of work is around physical health. There is currently a set of three *Healthy Body – Healthy Mind* resources available on the Shift website to help address physical health issues (http://www.shift.org.uk). These resources are aimed at service users, people working in inpatient services and people working in community-based services, with a further set for primary care practitioners being developed.

Research undertaken by the Joseph Rowntree Foundation looked at services for people with physical impairment and mental health needs and found that "inpatient experiences were often characterised by inaccessible physical environments and a lack of assistance for even simple things. There was a lack of understanding of the assistance that people needed, and staff were often too busy to provide it" (Morris, 2004).

A high proportion of wards (95%, 295 responses) reported that the CPA recorded some other special needs. This could include special dietary requirements, or relate to physical needs such as the use of a hoist for the bath etc.

Written treatment plan

Just over half the wards (55%, 302 responses) always had a written treatment plan produced within 72 hours. For most others, this was frequently the case. There were 28 wards nationally that only occasionally or rarely had a written treatment plan within 72 hours.

Carers

A national total of 99% (305 responses) of ward managers stated that service users could invite an advocate, carer and/or family members to care plan discussions, and that they were made aware of this. A total of 88% (299 responses) of ward managers reported that carers were named and noted in care plans.

Standard six of the NSF-MH states that more attention needs to be paid to carers and that:

"All individuals who provide regular and substantial care for a person on CPA should:

❖ Have an assessment of their caring, physical and mental health needs, repeated on at least an annual basis

❖ Have their own written care plan which is given to them and implemented in discussion with them."

(DH, 1999a)

Our findings show that 53% of ward managers reported that some carers of service users on their wards had their own care plans, but what our survey does not show is the overall number of carers with care plans. It may also be that some service users, when admitted to the ward, do not see their carers.

Figure 58   Wards where carers of patients on the wards have a written care plan for themselves (276 responses)

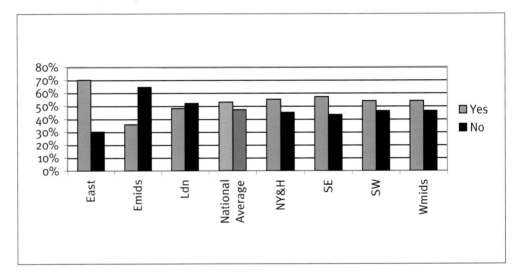

Crisis plans, advance directives and whole systems approach

Crisis plans should be drawn up as part of the care planning process to show staff, carers and service users what needs to be done if the service user experiences a mental health crisis. Crisis plans may be developed in the community or on a ward and we wanted to know whether ward staff have input into crisis plans developed in the community. We found that 55% of ward managers stated that they did.

Figure 59   Where crisis plans are developed in the community and inpatient care is identified do ward staff have input into the plan? (288 responses)

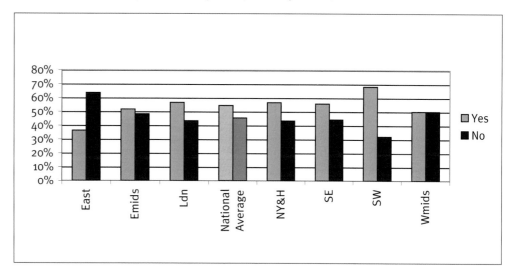

We then asked if wards had access to crisis plans developed in the community and we found considerable variation across and within regions. NY&H, West Midlands and South East regions showed the highest positive response at 79%, 70% and 63% respectively. The lowest figure was in Eastern region where only 27% of wards reported having access. London region showed marked differences between wards. Reviews of these survey findings by service users highlight this as an area of particular concern. Where time has been taken to develop these plans it is hoped that all staff would have access to them.

Figure 60   Do ward staff have access to crisis plans developed in the community? (287 responses)

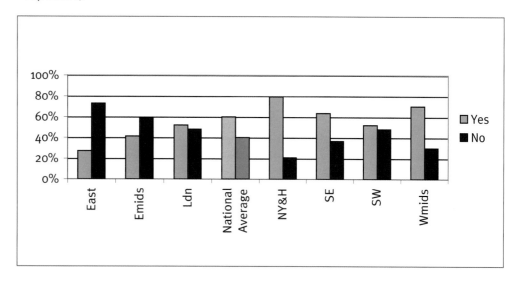

Advance directives are "a way of making a person's views known if he or she should become mentally incapable of giving consent to treatment, or making informed choices about treatment, at some future time" and would usually be made prior to hospital admission (http://www.mind.org.uk/Information/Legal/Legalbriefing+adv ancedirectives.htm). It may be that a service user does not want to be given a certain medication if he/she deteriorates and an advance directive is a way of ensuring that the doctors, nurses and others treating the service user are aware of this.

We do not know from this survey how widespread the use of advance directives is nationally, but less than half of ward managers reported that they had access to an advance directive where one had been drawn up by a service user. Only in NY&H was the percentage higher for those who had access at 53% compared to those who did not at 47%. This lack of access to advance directives is of concern and, as with crisis plans, indicates that for many trusts a whole systems approach to service user care is not happening.

Figure 61   Do ward staff have access to advance directives where drawn up by the service user? (285 responses)

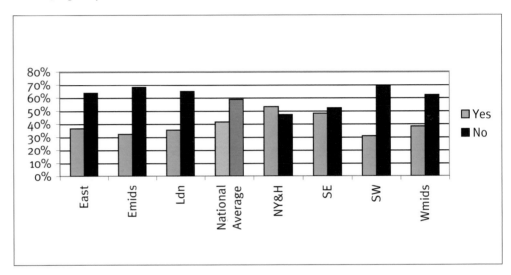

Where ward staff have access to crisis plans and advance directives, we wanted to know if there was a process which ensured that they were followed through. The findings show some regional variation, with only London and NY&H regions having a process in more than half of wards.

Figure 62   Is there a process which ensures crisis plans/advance directives are followed through? (273 responses)

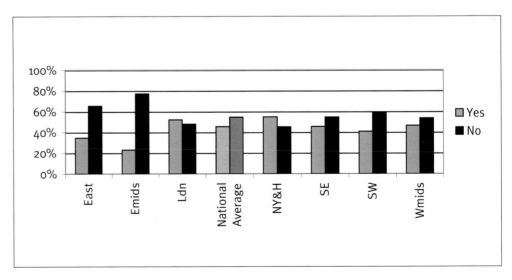

Admissions and discharge

Nationally, 87% of ward managers confirmed that CMHTs and GPs were notified of admissions and discharges within 72 hours. This is particularly high in London where 95% of wards confirmed that this does occur. It is of concern that nationally 13% of ward managers reported that CMHTs and GPs are not notified within 72 hours. This means that primary care and community services may not be aware that they need to take over care, and has implications for relapse and therefore re-admission rates.

Figure 63   Are GPs and CMHTs given details of all admissions and discharges within 72 hours of these occurring? (302 responses)

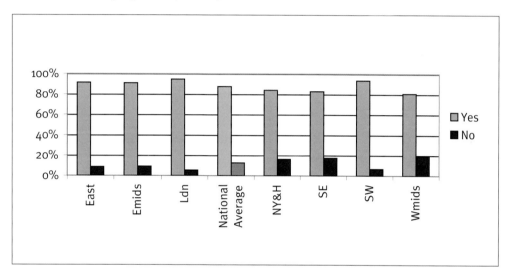

We wanted to know whether a representative from the CMHT always attended discharge planning meetings, and the most positive response was from London where 48% of ward managers reported this happening. Elsewhere in the country the figures drop to 30% or below. Figure 64 shows that there was considerable variation in the frequency of attendance within regions. A small number of wards in the East Midlands, Eastern, NY&H, South West and West Midlands regions reported that this rarely occurred, but they made up only 3% of wards. There may be a number of reasons why this was not occurring such as staff shortages or emergencies for the CMHT, or lack of adequate notice of meetings, or lack of a whole systems approach to care.

Figure 64   Does a representative from the CMHT attend discharge planning meetings? (306 responses)

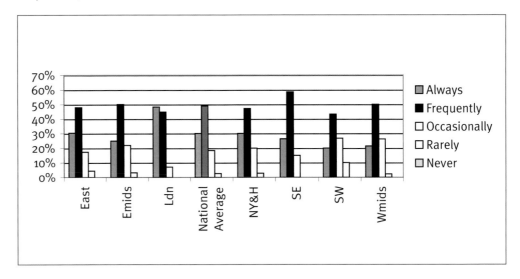

88% (306 responses) of ward managers confirmed that every client's CPA plan has written details of the involvement of all relevant agencies such as CMHTs at the time of discharge. Across all regions a small percentage of ward managers reported that this was not happening.

All these findings indicate that there is still more work to be done to facilitate improved communication between inpatient wards and community teams. Where new teams are setting up, such as crisis resolution teams (CRTs), it is essential that a whole systems approach to care is adopted to ensure that both wards and CRTs can function effectively and fulfil their remits.

RECOMMENDATIONS

CPA documentation   ❖ Trusts should ensure that there are clear local policies in place regarding the information required for CPA documentation which comply with Standard four of the NSF-MH (DH, 1999a).

❖ Trusts should ensure that when electronic CPA systems are implemented that documentation is streamlined to reduce the administrative workload and avoid repetition. It also needs to make key information easily accessible for all members of the multidisciplinary teams, both ward and community based.

Implementation   ❖ Trusts should use the Department of Health or CPAA audit tool annually to monitor the quality of CPA implementation.

❖ Ward managers should ensure that carers who meet the criteria of Standard Six of the NSF-MH have had both an initial assessment and a care plan drawn up. Where this has not happened, the appropriate action should be taken in liaison with the CPA care co-ordinator.

Crisis plans/
advance directives   ❖ Trusts/ACFs should investigate why ward staff are not gaining access to crisis plans and advance directives drawn up in the community and to ensure systems are put in place to address this.

❖ Trusts/education providers should look at designing multidisciplinary training workshops on the use of crisis plans and advance directives.

❖ Trusts/ACFs/ward managers/consultant psychiatrists/pharmacists and other members of the multidisciplinary team should look at establishing processes for following crisis plans and advance directives.

Whole systems approach

❖ Trusts should enable systems to be put in place to ensure that community teams and GPs are notified of service user admission and discharge at least within 72 hours. Any system needs to be simple and should avoid the creation of administrative burden for frontline staff.

❖ Trusts should follow Adult Acute MH-PIG suggestions on setting operational policies that take a whole systems approach to building services that are part of an integrated system.

Positive practice

❖ RDCs should facilitate the dissemination of positive practice in any of the above areas within and across regions

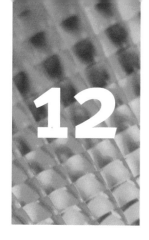

12 Environment

"Poor standards of design, lack of space and access to basic amenities and comforts in much of our current inpatient provision have contributed to and reinforced service users' negative experiences of inpatient care as unsafe, uncomfortable and untherapeutic."

Mental Health Policy Implementation Guide:
Adult Acute Inpatient Care Provision (DH, 2002a)

KEY FINDINGS

❖ 78% of ward managers stated that the ward did promote positive mental health care

❖ 82% of ward managers reported that cleanliness on the ward was satisfactory

❖ 34% of ward managers stated that there were significant reported but unresolved environmental risks on the ward

❖ 64% of ward managers reported that where ward areas/facilities needed repair that this was carried out promptly

❖ 61% of ward managers had access to the £5,000 ward environment budget for making local improvements and there were significant regional differences in access to this fund

❖ 86% of ward managers confirmed that service users were consulted about the quality of the environment

❖ Service users could control lighting on most wards but not temperature

❖ Just over half the wards had sufficient quiet areas for service users but less than half had sufficient quiet areas for service users to meet with friends and relatives

❖ A small number of wards did not have separate sleeping areas, bathrooms and toilets for men and women

❖ Most service users had private access to a phone and could bring mobile phones into hospital but email access was limited

❖ 80% of wards had unrestricted access to hot and cold drinks and food

CONTEXT

In 2003 the *Health Service Journal* launched its 'Fit for Purpose' campaign "demanding urgent action to improve the depressing and dangerous environments in which many service users are still treated". Mental health trust performance ratings for 2004/5 include 'physical environment' which looks at "environmental conditions, space relationships, service effectiveness, amenity, and location all of which impact on the successful delivery of client care" and the rating categories range from 'A' ("very satisfactory, no change needed") to category 'X' which indicates that "nothing but a total rebuild or relocation will suffice" (http://ratings2004.healthcarecommission.org.uk).

Patient Environment Action Teams (PEAT) assess cleanliness and other aspects of the patient environment and score hospitals using a 5-point scale. The PEAT programme commenced in 2000 and assessments are undertaken on an annual basis to ensure that standards are being met (http://www.cleanhospitals.com).

The need for the building of new inpatient units was identified in *Not Just Bricks and Mortar* but the report recognised that there is no formulaic solution to the problems of planning and constructing these new builds. The report makes a number of recommendations that take into account size, staffing, structure, siting and security as "these dimensions are mutually dependent and impact each other directly" (Royal College of Psychiatrists, 1998a).

In 1999 the NHS Executive published *Safety, privacy and dignity in mental health units: Guidance on mixed sex accommodation for mental health services* which also looks at a range of issues including design. The provision of single sex accommodation has proved to be a contentious issue. In June 2004 Minister of State for Health, Rosie Winterton, reported to the House of Commons that "99 per cent of all NHS trusts provided single-sex sleeping accommodation for planned admissions" and that "97 per cent of all NHS trusts provided properly segregated bathroom and toilet facilities for men and women". However in Mind's *Ward Watch* survey (2004) 23% of respondents reported having recently been or that they were currently in mixed sex wards and 31% of respondents said they did not have the use of single sex bathrooms.

NHS Estates has recently funded research that looked at "the effect of the hospital environment on the patient experience and health outcomes" and they found that "in the mental health sector patient treatment times were reduced by 14%" as a result of the new accommodation (http://patientexperience.nhsestates.gov.uk/healing_environment/he_content/home/home.asp). In February 2000 the King's Fund launched its 'Enhancing the Healing Environment Programme'. Due to its success with acute care trusts, they have expanded the programme to include mental health trusts in London that will have nurse-led teams working with service users to look at ways to improve the environment. The London HAS report (2003) stated that the new builds visits during their benchmarking "were impressive" and that "in addition to the high priority given to patient safety, the new builds enhance the working conditions of staff". They also found "examples of good refurbishment to old premises where new builds were not viable" and that key to these "was a

strong link between estates and facilities, service manager and ward managers"
(HAS, 2003).

WHAT WE FOUND

Our survey looked at general issues concerning the environment and then more specifically at the service user and the ward environment.

Promotion of positive mental health care

The Mind survey (2004) found that 53% of current or recent inpatients, who responded, felt that the ward environment had not helped their recovery. By contrast, when we asked ward managers if the environment on the ward promoted positive mental health care we found that 78% of ward managers believed that it did.

Figure 65   Does the environment promote positive mental health care for service users? (298 responses)

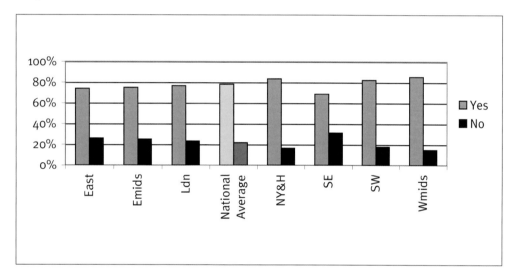

Ward environment budget

The ward environment budget of £5,000 was set up to enable ward managers to "best enhance and humanise patient care or improve the working lives of staff" (http://www.purchasingcard.nhs.uk/introduction/index.asp). In 2001 ward managers were allocated £5,000 and purchase cards were developed. In the House of Commons on 6 May 2004 it was reported that "it was for decision by individual NHS trusts whether to join the scheme and to issue cards to ward managers. As at April 2004, there are 2,000 purchase cards being used in the NHS". NHS Estates advise that where trusts decide not to issue these funds, they are expected to agree this course of action with their strategic health authority.

Our survey shows that only 61% of ward managers stated that they had access to this budget, leaving over a third of managers without access. Figure 66 shows the considerable regional variation in access to this budget.

Figure 66   Does the ward manager have access to the £5,000 ward environment budget to make local improvements? (293 responses)

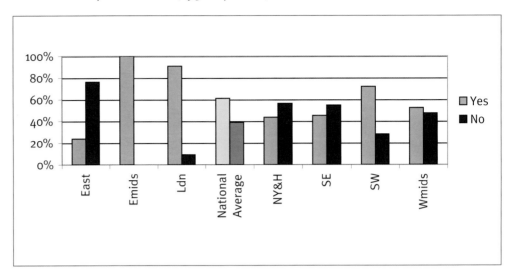

Unresolved environmental risks and repairs   We asked if there were any significant reported but unresolved environmental risks on the ward and 34% of ward managers stated that there were. This survey did not seek to identify what those risks were and this would need to be undertaken as part of any local review.

Figure 67   Are there any significant reported but unresolved environmental risks on the ward? (301 responses)

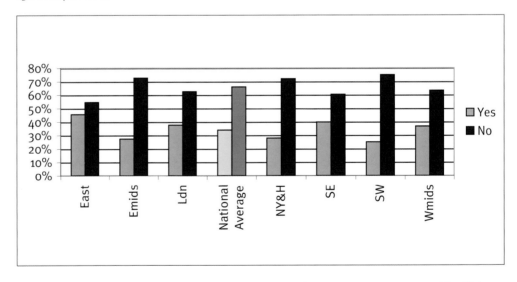

We found that 64% of ward managers confirmed that repairs to areas and facilities were carried out promptly. However, this does leave 36% of ward managers reporting that repairs were not carried out quickly and this may in part be related to the percentage of reported but unresolved risks.

Figure 68   In general if areas or facilities require repair are these carried out quickly? (304 responses)

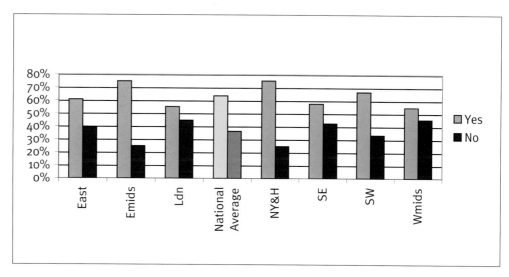

Floor and level of the ward in the building   To gain a picture of where acute inpatient wards were placed within a hospital setting we asked which floor the ward was based on. In most regions the majority of wards were on the ground floor. London is the exception to this with the majority of wards based on the first floor or above and only 20% of wards on the ground floor. Possible reasons for this include pressure of space and land costs. The ideal is to have the ward on the ground floor thus giving service users easy access to fresh air, exercise and recreation in a safe and managed way. Furthermore, the risk of harm to people who may jump from upper floors either to abscond or commit suicide would be eliminated by ground floor provision.

Figure 69   What floor in the building is the ward on? (303 responses)

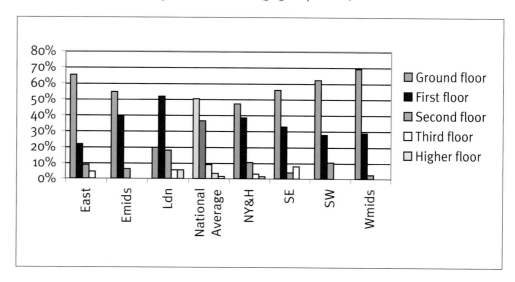

We also wanted to know if the ward was based on one floor or whether it was split. There are implications for the staffing levels of wards split over more than one floor, as this may present difficulties in the general observation of service users. Nationally, 22 ward managers (7%) reported that their ward was divided over more than one floor. The highest percentage of wards split over more than one floor was 12%, in the NY&H region.

Cleanliness and décor

We asked about the general cleanliness of the wards and nationally, 82% of ward managers stated that this was satisfactory. The range of positive responses ranged from 77% in the South West to 90% in the West Midlands.

We asked about the overall décor of the ward and 72% of ward managers reported that this was satisfactory. The positive responses ranged here from 64% in the East Midlands to 81% in the West Midlands.

Consultation with service users

We asked if service users were consulted about the quality of the ward environment. We found that 86% of ward managers confirmed that service users were consulted and in the South West all ward managers who took part in the survey confirmed this happened.

Outdoor space and daylight

Nationally, a total of 79% of ward managers reported that service users had access to a suitable outdoor space. However, in the East Midlands region this dropped to 61% of wards with 13 wards in the region reporting that there was no suitable outdoor space.

Figure 70   Do service users have access to a suitable outdoor space? (304 responses)

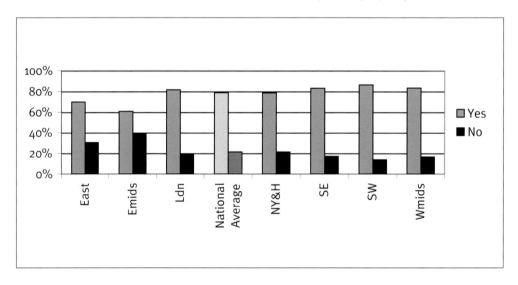

The survey shows that on most wards (93%) service users' rooms had natural daylight. However it is worrying that 22 ward managers (7%) who took part in the survey reported that service users' rooms did not have natural daylight.

Controlling the ward environment – lighting, heating, smoking

Similarly 91% of ward managers reported that service users were able to control the lighting. However this still leaves 28 wards where ward managers reported service users could not control lighting.

Results were more disappointing in terms of service users being able to control environmental temperature such as adjusting heating. Only 17% of ward managers reported that service users could control the temperature. Across the regions percentages ranged from 6% in the East Midlands to 19% in NY&H, South East and West Midlands regions.

Only four ward managers (1%) reported there were not clearly defined smoking and non-smoking areas. These wards were in East Midlands, London and NY&H regions. This number of wards is very small but the risks of passive smoking are well documented and it is of concern that service users on these wards are subjected to this health risk while in hospital.

Quiet areas   We asked whether there were sufficient quiet areas for service users and 54% of ward managers stated that there were.

Figure 71   Are there sufficient quiet areas for service users? (306 responses)

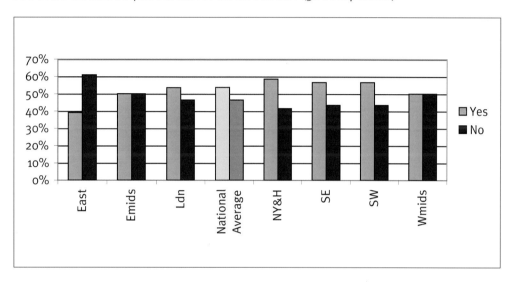

Nationally, less than half of ward managers (46%) stated that there were sufficient areas for service users to spend quiet time with relatives or friends. In the Eastern region 19 ward managers (83%) reported that there were not sufficient areas.

Children visiting   Nationally, 65% of ward managers stated that safe facilities were provided for children visiting the ward. There were some regional differences, with this figure rising to 84% in NY&H and dropping to 48% in the West Midlands.

Figure 72   Are there safe facilities provided for children visiting the ward? (301 responses)

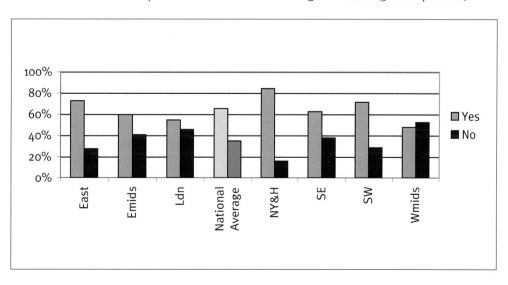

Shared accommodation

Where shared accommodation still exists, we wanted to find out some detail about how these facilities were managed. However, there appeared to be data quality issues with the responses to these questions and difficulties in defining shared accommodation, so we were unable to ascertain with certainty the number of wards which have shared accommodation. What we can present is findings on the numbers of wards without separate sleeping areas, bathrooms and toilets for men and women.

Sleeping areas

We found that a total of 25 ward managers reported that they did not have separate sleeping areas for men and women. These were found across all regions with the exception of East Midlands. We can only calculate an estimated percentage based on the maximum number of wards that took part in the survey as opposed to the actual number that responded to the question. Based on this, it would mean that 8% of wards did not have separate sleeping areas.

Bathrooms

A total of 26 ward managers reported that they did not have separate bathrooms for men and women. These were across all the regions.

Toilets

A total of 11 ward managers reported that they did not have separate toilets for men and women. These were in all regions except the East Midlands and the East.

Service user property, telephone and email access

There were appropriate arrangements for the safekeeping of service users' property on 92% of wards. However, 17% of wards in the Eastern region and 15% of wards in the South East did not have that facility.

There was private access to a telephone for service users on 81% of wards and again most wards allowed service users to bring in a mobile phone (86%).

Private email access for service users was very limited with only 42 ward managers (14%) reporting that this facility was offered on their ward. Wards with private email access were found throughout the regions with the exception of East Midlands.

Refreshments

The *Mental Health Policy Implementation Guide: Adult Acute Inpatient Care Provision* (MH-PIG Adult Acute) states that "service users should have access to drinks and refreshments at all times" and 80% of wards confirmed that they did (DH, 2002a). However, this still leaves 61 wards with restricted access.

We asked whether foods for special dietary requirements were readily available and found that 96% of ward managers confirmed that they were.

RECOMMENDATIONS

Identifying problems / areas for change

❖ Trusts need to identify where the problem areas are for acute inpatient wards, particularly those 22% of wards where ward managers stated that the ward environment did not promote positive mental health care. Problems may be general such as overall shabbiness or more specific such as overcrowded smoking rooms. Ward staff, service users, carers and visitors should be involved in identifying the problem areas.

❖ Trusts should look carefully at refurbishment and other changes in order to create an ambience of calm and comfort and reduce risk. Staff, service users, carers and visitors should be consulted on any proposed changes.

❖ Ward managers should report all unresolved risks to the Acute Care Forum, which will in turn report this through the clinical governance structure. This is to ensure that the trust board is aware of the issues and that plans are put in place to manage and resolve the risks within a given time frame. Ward managers should be kept informed of proposed plans and time frames.

Guidance

❖ Trusts/wards should follow *Safety, privacy and dignity in mental health units: guidance on mixed sex accommodation for mental health services* (NHS Executive, 2000), the MH-PIG Adult Acute (DH, 2002a) and should also look at the recommendations in *Not Just Bricks and Mortar* (Royal College of Psychiatrists, 1999a).

❖ Trusts need to assess and prioritise space and room allocation to meet the requirements set out in the guidance.

Housekeepers

❖ Trusts/modern matrons should consider appointing ward housekeepers who could take a central role in monitoring the cleanliness, décor and speed of necessary repairs. NHS Estates provides information on the housekeeper role.

Service user needs and choice

❖ Trusts/modern matrons/ward managers should look at ways in which service user control of the environment can be improved, such as the ability to control temperature and lighting. Where ward managers have access to the ward environment budget, this may be an area where the money could be used.

❖ Modern matrons/ward managers should review current practices around the restriction of hot and cold drinks.

❖ Trusts need to take action regarding the very small number of wards that do not have clear smoking and non-smoking areas. The health risks associated with smoking and passive smoking are well documented and service users who do not wish to smoke must have a clear non-smoking area.

❖ NHS Estates/modern matrons/ward managers should look at how access to private telephones can be improved on the wards.

Ward environment budget

❖ NHS Estates/strategic health authorities should review why some trusts are not allocating the ward environment budget to the ward manager, most notably in the East, NY&H and South East. The implications of ward managers not having the budget should be looked into.

❖ Trusts should provide ward managers who are not given the ward environment budget with clear mechanisms for gaining access to funding to improve the ward environment.

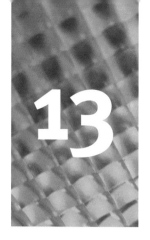

13 Therapies and activities

"Inpatient units that provide appropriate stimulation and structure as part of individual care plans have a more therapeutic and safe environment. Yet a recurring theme in most reports on inpatient care is 'lack of something to do' (as one report puts it 'a sort of suspended animation')."

Mental Health Policy Implementation Guide: Adult Acute Inpatient Care Provision (DH, 2002a)

KEY FINDINGS

❖ Social and leisure activities were routinely available on 64% of wards

❖ Practical therapeutic activities were routinely available on 73% of wards

❖ Despite their clear evidence base, neither cognitive behavioural therapy nor psychosocial interventions were routinely available on most inpatient wards

❖ Ward managers reported that nurses and occupational therapists provide the largest percentage input into activities/therapies

❖ Less than a quarter of ward managers reported having input from psychologists into therapies/activities

CONTEXT

The report *What CHI has found in mental health trusts* stated that boredom was a common problem for service users on wards (Healthcare Commission, 2003). This can be exacerbated when staff shortages and usage of agency staff result in a reduced number of activities offered to service users. CHI reported that service users often said that "the range and quality of activities are limited" (Healthcare Commission, 2003). This finding is not new. *Acute Problems* reported that as many as 30% of service users said that they were not involved in any therapeutic or recreational activity at all during their hospital stay (SCMH, 1998). Apart from mental well being, the potential impact of boredom on physical health is highlighted in *Not all in the Mind* (mentality, 2003). This report identifies a 'smoking culture' on psychiatric wards whereby smoking, with its known health risks, becomes a means to alleviate boredom and to provide social interaction.

A recent ethnographic study carried out by the Royal College of Psychiatrists suggests that service user complaints of not having someone to talk to "can largely be explained by the centrality of medication, the limited availability of talking therapy, and the passing relationships users have with nurses" (Quirk & Lelliott, 2004).

In this survey we aimed to obtain an overview of the range and type of activities that were available on the wards. We have categorised these into:

❖ social and leisure activities

❖ practical therapeutic activities

❖ talking therapies

We also examined the types of specific therapeutic approaches, for example art therapy, and asked who was providing or conducting ward activities.

WHAT WE FOUND

Social and leisure activities could include going to the gym, coffee mornings, bingo, karaoke evenings etc. We found that social and leisure activities were routinely available on 195 wards (64%) and were occasionally available on 31% of wards but not available at all on 5% of wards. This means that on almost 40% of wards in England, social and leisure activities were only occasionally available, or not available at all: a high figure when it is considered that these types of activities can be developed by any member of the team or by volunteers.

Practical therapeutic activities include learning cooking skills, developing skills in organising finances and art therapy, and 73% of ward managers report that these were routinely provided. However, they were not available at all on 2% of wards.

Talking therapies include a range of different therapies such as cognitive behavioural therapy (CBT), psychotherapy, psychosocial interventions etc. but from our findings, there seems to be some issue around the definition of talking therapies. Some ward managers may have included the use of counselling skills/ talking with service users, which although therapeutic, do not fall into one of the recognised formal therapeutic interventions, such as CBT. Other ward managers may have only included these specific therapies. It is therefore with caution that we present the findings for talking therapies. We found that 73% of ward managers reported that talking therapies were routinely available but 4% of ward managers reported that no talking therapy was available on their wards.

Figure 73   National breakdown of activities available on the wards (310 responses)

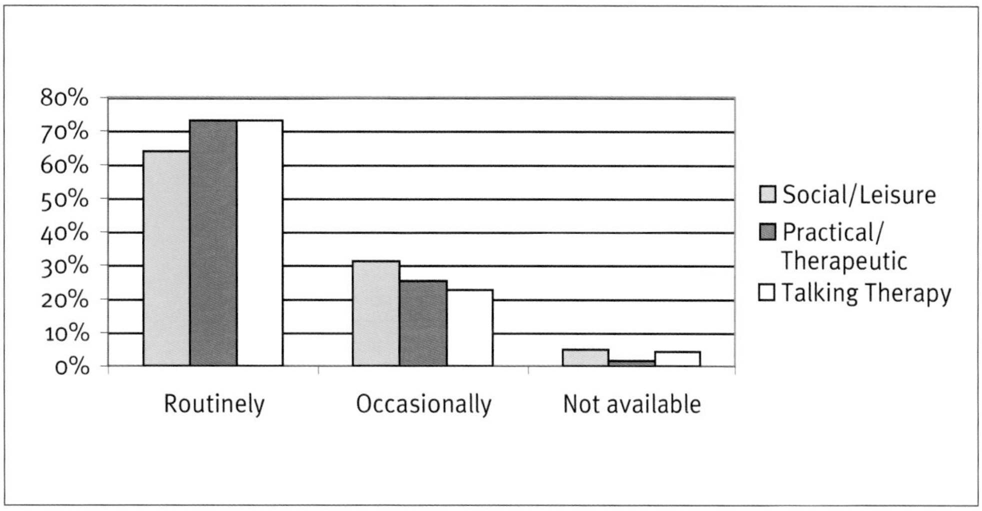

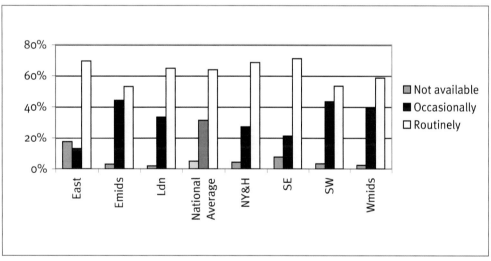

We have analysed each category of activity by region. The South East had the highest percentage of wards where leisure and social activities were routinely available at 71%. East Midlands and the South West both had the lowest rate, at 53%.

Figure 74   How often are leisure and social activities available on the ward? (304 responses)

We have analysed each category of activity by region. The South East had the highest percentage of wards where leisure and social activities were routinely available at 71%. East Midlands and the South West both had the lowest rate, at 53%.

For practical therapeutic activities, the average percentages for routine availability range from 50% in the East Midlands to 83% in the South West (see Figure 75).

Figure 75   How often are practical therapies available on the ward? (308 responses)

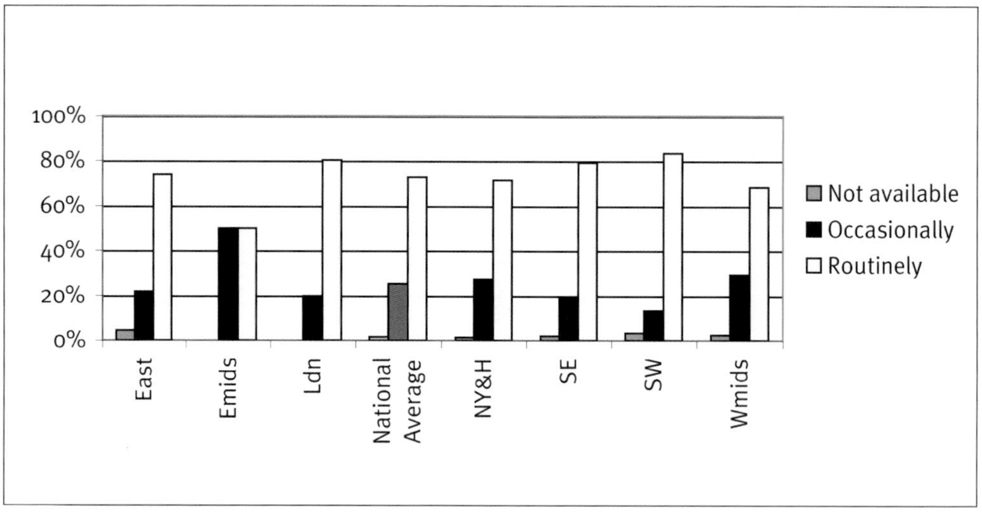

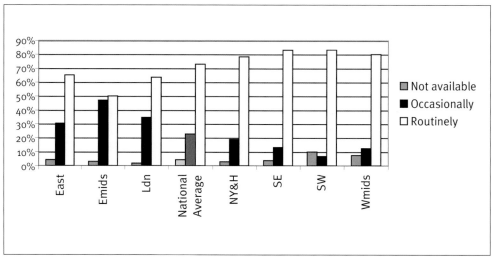

We found that the range of availability of talking therapies varied from 50% at the lowest, in the East Midlands region, and 83% at the highest, in the South West and South East. However, as previously stated, there may have been different interpretations of talking therapies, which could have affected these regional findings.

Figure 76   How often are talking therapy activities available on the ward? (304 responses)

Specific therapies   We found that the most common routinely available therapy was art therapy but that its availability was not consistent across all wards. Our survey results show that 49% of ward managers reported having art therapy routinely available with a further 31% of wards offering this occasionally. However, art therapy was not available at all on 20% of wards.

Ward managers reported that the second most routinely available therapeutic approach was psychosocial interventions at 35%. Despite their strong evidence base, cognitive behavioural therapy (CBT), solution focused behavioural therapy and family therapy were only routinely available on fewer than 20% of wards. Such interventions do require a level of training that is often unavailable or not accessible to ward staff and it may not always be appropriate to conduct these therapies whilst the service user is in a disturbed state. When such training is undertaken the support and time to practise these skills is often not available (Clarke, 2004).

Figure 77 Availability of specific therapeutic approaches available for service users on the ward (310 responses)

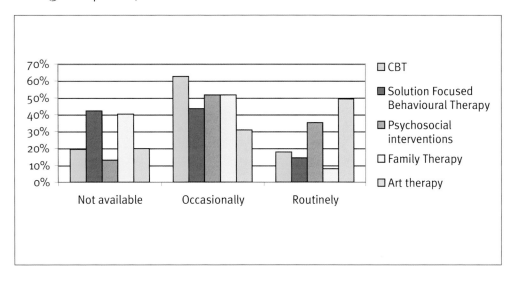

Multidisciplinary approach

The *Mental Health Policy Implementation Guide: Adult Acute Inpatient Care Provision* considers that a "key factor contributing to a sense of boredom and lack of service user engagement on inpatient wards is inadequate clinical input for the ward from the full range of care professions that comprise the mental health multidisciplinary team" (DH, 2002a). *Acute Problems* highlighted a lack of multidisciplinary input, stating that contact with staff other than nurses and doctors was minimal (SCMH, 1998).

In our survey, we looked specifically at activities and therapies and therefore these findings do not include types of input to service user care such as ward reviews. Ward managers reported that nurses and OTs were providing the bulk of input into service user activities/therapies on the ward. Figure 78 shows that 13% of ward managers reported having input from medical staff, 23% from psychologists and 35% from other staff (such as therapists, activity workers, health care assistants etc.).

Figure 78 Staff groups that ward managers reported have input into service user activities/ therapies on the ward (310 responses)

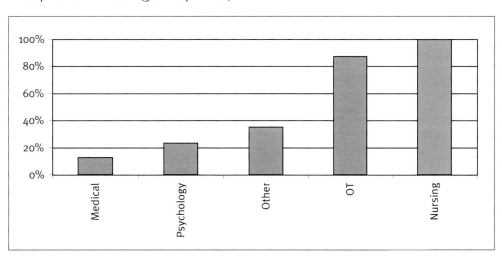

There was regional variation with medical (psychiatrist) input ranging from 6% in the South East to 17% in the South West and psychologist input ranging from 3% of wards in the East Midlands to 35% in the Eastern region. This raises the question of how much and what type of input into activities/therapies is required from psychiatrists and psychologists and whether the current input into activities is adequate to meet the needs of the service users and fulfil the requirements of policy implementation guidance.

RECOMMENDATIONS

Promoting activities

❖ Trusts should acknowledge the important role of activities in service users' recovery by ensuring that staff are given planned and protected time to make sure activities are provided regularly and routinely. The frequency, regularity and diversity of activities should be monitored.

❖ Trust/ACFs/RDCs should ensure that positive practice is shared.

Training

❖ Trusts should adopt a systematic whole ward, multidisciplinary team training approach to enable culture and practice to change.

❖ Trusts should increase the availability of training and practice development related to evidence based approaches such as CBT. They need also to take measures to ensure that inpatient staff are encouraged, enabled and supported to get this training/practice development and then given the opportunity to practise once trained.

Multidisciplinary approach

❖ Trusts should consider clarifying the role of qualified nursing staff in providing ward activities in line with current professional guidance.

❖ Trusts need to increase the psychology time (and/or psychotherapy time) available to inpatient units both to facilitate training and to increase the delivery of psychological interventions to service users on the wards

❖ Trusts need to explore the involvement of HCAs, volunteers, sessional workers, and activity workers in facilitating a broader range and availability of activities. Opportunities must be afforded for staff to develop their motivational and engagement skills.

❖ NIMHE and the Royal College of Psychiatrists are currently carrying out work to consider the role of psychiatrists in providing acute inpatient care. Trusts should consider how to achieve their integration as members of multidisciplinary ward teams. Greater engagement with service users and practitioners would support this process.

Regional variation

❖ RDCs should work in partnership with trusts and ACFs, drawing their attention to the Adult Acute MH-PIG regarding activities, in order to identify the reasons for the different type and level of activities available across the regions. This should act as a prompt for ACFs to take appropriate remedial action.

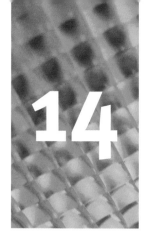

14 Equality issues

"Values need to be translated into appropriate practice, structure and relationships that promote human and therapeutic inpatient care in the overall context of continuing service improvement."

Mental Health Policy Implementation Guide: Adult Acute Inpatient Care Provision (DH, 2002a)

KEY FINDINGS

❖ 55% of wards had a policy with regard to cultural sensitivity

❖ 26% of ward managers reported that none of their staff had training with regard to cultural sensitivity

❖ 8% of ward managers reported that their ward uses a cultural sensitivity audit tool

❖ 96% of ward managers confirmed that there was adequate access to interpreting facilities for people from minority ethnic groups

❖ 62% of ward managers reported that there was adequate access to professionals from similar backgrounds for people from minority ethnic groups

❖ 97% of ward managers confirmed that female service users had adequate access to women staff at all times

❖ 64% of ward managers reported that they either partially or fully met the needs of people with sensory impairment

❖ 87% of ward managers reported that there was access throughout the ward, including toilets and bathrooms, for people with mobility difficulties

CONTEXT

The *NHS Plan* states that "services will be available when people require them, tailored to their individual needs" (DH, 2000a). *Acute Inpatient Mental Health Care: Education, Training & Continuing Professional Development for All* states that staff need to be able to "respect diversity, acknowledge similarities across cultures and confront discriminatory practices" (Clarke, 2004). Some groups can be less likely to have their individual needs met and these include people from minority ethnic groups, women and people with sensory/physical impairment.

In September 2004, The Joseph Rowntree Foundation published findings on *Experiencing ethnicity: Discrimination and service provision,* showing "the persistence of racist experiences, inadequate support and service responses to meet the diversity of need, and the continued need for recognising diversity within and between minority ethnic groups" (Chalal & Ullah, 2004). Earlier work carried out by the Sainsbury Centre for Mental Health highlighted the particular problems facing African and Caribbean service users (SCMH, 2002). *Inside Outside: Improving Mental Health Services for Black and Minority Ethnic Communities in England* aims to set out "three key objectives and recommendations" for achieving change to improve services (DH, 2003a) and *Engaging and Changing: Developing effective policy for the care and treatment of Black and minority ethnic detained patients* was produced to assist in the development of policies (NIMHE, 2003a). *Delivering Race Equality in Mental Health Care: An action plan for reform inside and outside services and the Government's response to the independent inquiry into the death of David Bennett* (DRE) was published by the Department of Health in January 2005 and "sets out a clear action plan for achieving equality and eradicating unlawful discrimination in mental health services in England". In our survey we have asked some questions to find out about issues relating largely to cultural awareness on the acute inpatient ward.

Issues specifically affecting women are raised in the *Mental Health Policy Implementation Guide: Adult Acute Inpatient Care Provision* (MH-PIG Adult Acute) (DH, 2002a) and again in more detail in *Mainstreaming Gender and Women's Mental Health: Implementation Guidance* (DH, 2003b). This guidance makes it clear that "all organisations should aim to ensure that they are sensitive to gender (and ethnicity) and the specific needs of women". In our survey we did not aim to cover this topic fully. Some of our findings are specifically related to environmental issues and are found in the environment chapter. Here we have selected one element of the MH-PIG Adult Acute to survey which relates to female service users' access to female staff.

The Joseph Rowntree Foundation recently published the findings of research which explored "services for people with physical impairments and mental health support needs" (Morris, 2004). The research found that "two-thirds of respondents said they had difficulty accessing mental health services because of their physical impairment" and the report highlights a number of serious concerns including the withdrawal of pain relief needed for physical conditions upon admission to psychiatric wards (Morris, 2004). The *Department of Health/Disability Rights Commission framework for partnership action on disability 2004/5* states that the "Department of Health is committed to patient and user-centred services which are equitable and accessible for all and which underpin disabled people's social inclusion in other areas of life" (DH & DRC, 2004). In our survey we asked a number of questions to find out how sensitive services are to people with physical impairment.

WHAT WE FOUND

Cultural sensitivity Nationally, 163 ward managers (55%) reported having a policy with regard to cultural sensitivity. A further 16% of ward managers reported that a policy was being developed.

Figure 79 Does the ward have a policy with regard to cultural sensitivity? (297 responses)

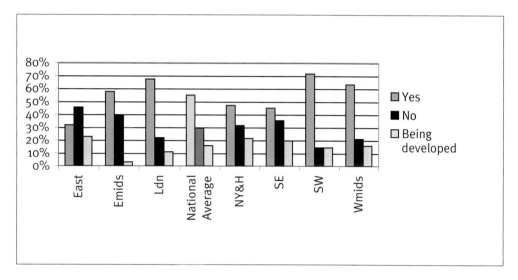

Only eight ward managers reported that all staff had undertaken training regarding cultural sensitivity. Those ward managers were based in London, West Midlands and NY&H regions. Although high percentages of ward managers reported that either some staff (56%) or most staff (16%) had undertaken training, some 26% of ward managers reported that none of the staff had undertaken training in cultural sensitivity. As Figure 80 shows, there was a considerable range of responses within each region.

Figure 80 How many of the ward staff have had training regarding cultural sensitivity? (302 responses)

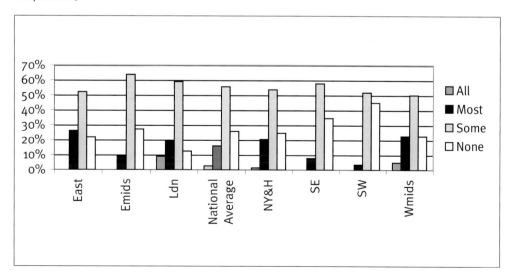

The Sainsbury Centre for Mental Health developed the *Cultural Sensitivity Audit Tool for Mental Health Services*. Its aim is "to help mental health services evaluate their current strengths and weaknesses by identifying the context in which the service is provided, learning from the experiences of service users and of staff, and putting all of this together to form an action plan for change" (Sathyamoorthy *et al.,* 2001). This audit tool is being revised and updated. Other cultural sensitivity audit tools may have been created locally. We wanted to find out how many wards were using some form of audit tool. Only 8% of ward managers reported using a cultural sensitivity audit tool and regional use varies from 3% in the South West and East Midlands to 13% in London and West Midlands.

The report *Real Voices* identified language as one of six key issues "contributing to ethnic minority disadvantage with mental health services" (NIMHE, 2003b). *Delivering Race Equality* also highlights this problem and states that "NIMHE has convened a national group ... to develop best practice guidance on interpreting, translation and communication support with mental health settings" (DH, 2005), with a report due to be available in 2005.

We found that 96% (299 responses) of ward managers felt that there was adequate access to interpreting facilities for people from minority ethnic groups. Our survey findings are therefore at odds with the reports detailed above and it is important to note that our findings relate solely to ward managers' perceptions of these facilities and do not include the views of service users.

Delivering Race Equality states that "the mental health workforce needs to become representative of the population at all levels" (DH, 2005). Nationally, 62% of ward managers reported that there was adequate access to professionals from similar backgrounds for people from minority ethnic groups. A total of 6% of wards were not able to answer this question suggesting that there may be uncertainty about what is deemed adequate or about the ethnic diversity of the ward during the previous 12 months. The latter is reflected in the 2002/3 Hospital Episode Statistics where 15 – 26% of service users had not had their ethnicity recorded.

Figure 81 Does the ward have adequate access to professionals from similar backgrounds for people from minority ethnic groups? (309 responses)

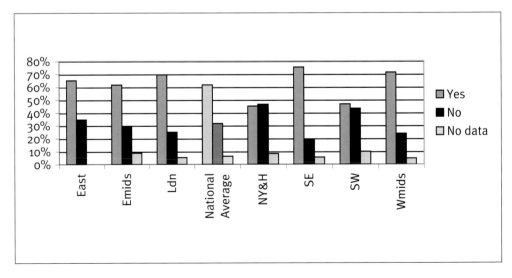

The majority of ward managers (92%) reported that there was adequate pastoral/spiritual support for people from minority ethnic groups and this was 100% in the East Midlands. All other regions report small percentages without adequate pastoral/spiritual support.

Women   The MH-PIG Adult Acute states that "staffing arrangements need to ensure women have adequate access to women staff at all times, particularly with regard to choice of keyworkers, control and restraint, physical health care and counselling" (DH, 2002a). We wanted to know if ward managers felt that female service users have adequate access to women staff at all times. We found that 97% of ward managers confirmed that this was the case. In the South West this figure is 100%. A total of eight wards spread across the other regions reported that this was not the case.

Sensory impairment   We asked if the ward fully met the needs of people with sensory impairments and only 6% of ward managers stated this was the case for their ward. However, 58% of ward managers reported that the ward partially meets the needs of people with sensory impairment. There still remained 109 ward managers (36%) who reported that their wards did not meet those needs at all and those wards were found across all regions.

Figure 82   Does the ward meet the needs of people with sensory impairment? (304 responses)

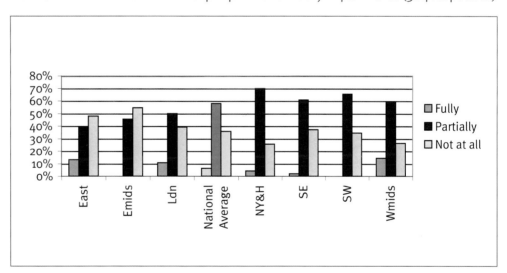

It is not surprising therefore to find that 137 ward managers (46%) reported that the range of dedicated mental health information for people with sensory impairment was poor (46%) and a further 17% reported that it was very poor. Of the remaining ward managers, 27% stated this was fair, 9% good and 1% excellent. Those with an excellent range of dedicated mental health information were found in Eastern, NY&H and South West regions.

Figure 83   How good is the range of dedicated mental health information for people with sensory impairments? (300 responses)

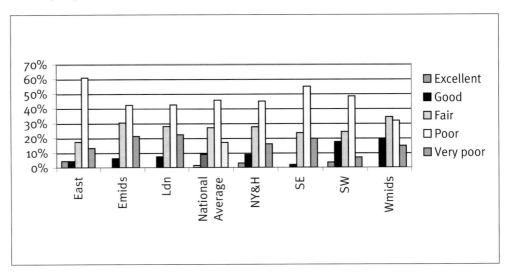

Mobility difficulties   Nationally, 87% of ward managers stated that there was access throughout the wards, including toilets and bathrooms, for people with mobility problems. However, it is of concern that 13% of ward managers reported that there was inadequate access.

Special equipment   We asked about ease of access to special equipment. For those with mobility problems, for example, this could include bath hoists and other lifting equipment. We found that 61% of ward managers stated that it was easy to get access to special equipment but in London this percentage dropped down to 35%. It is not clear why this may be lower in London and this would require local review.

Figure 84   Is it easy to get access to special equipment? (299 responses)

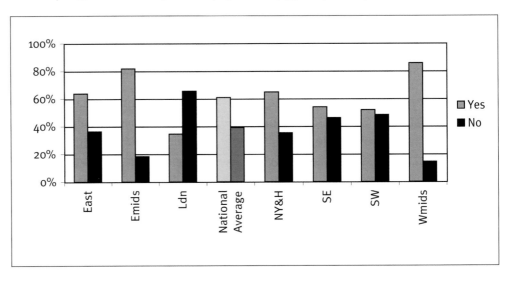

RECOMMENDATIONS

Service user views on equality

❖ Trusts should gather anonymised service user views on all these equality issues in order to inform service improvements.

Race equality

❖ Trusts should implement the recommendations in *Breaking the Circles of Fear* (SCMH, 2002), *Delivering Race Equality* (DH, 2005) and also *Mental Health Services Workforce Design and Development* (DH, 2003c).

❖ NIMHE race equality and acute care leads/fellows should use the findings of this report to inform programmes of work relating to race equality and acute inpatient care within their regions and/or nationally.

Training

❖ Trusts should provide mandatory training for all staff on issues of ethnicity, culture and racism and this should be part of a broader strategy for achieving race equality.

❖ Trusts should ensure that staff have disability awareness and disability equality training.

Women staff

❖ Ward managers/modern matrons should inform the acute care forum (ACF) if a ward does not offer adequate access to women staff for women service users (particularly key workers) as per the policy guidance. This can be reported by the ACF to the trust board as appropriate.

Service users with sensory/physical impairment

❖ The Department of Health should consult with specialist charities and organisations (e.g. The Royal National Institute for Deaf People) on how to make services accessible for people with sensory or physical impairments.

❖ RDCs should collect and disseminate positive practice with regard to dedicated mental health information for those with sensory impairment. This information could be posted on the NIMHE Knowledge Community.

❖ NHS Estates/trusts should assess environmental factors such as wheelchair access and other environmental factors for those with physical impairment/ disability.

❖ ACFs should assess the provision of special equipment within their trust and ensure that unmet need is reported to the trust management. Wards also need to be given clear guidelines on how to access special equipment for people with any form of physical impairment.

Policies

❖ Trusts should ensure that all staff are aware of and are implementing local and national policies on equality issues.

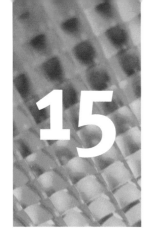

15 Acute Care Forums

"Each NHS Trust must establish an Acute Care Forum, with links across the elements of the acute care system (to include intensive care) and with involvement of service users and carers to agree and regularly review the operation and co-ordination of the range of acute care."

Mental Health Policy Implementation Guide:
Adult Acute Inpatient Care Provision (DH, 2002a)

KEY FINDINGS

❖ 94% of ward managers confirmed that there was an Acute Care Forum in their trust

❖ 88% of ward managers thought that they could influence their Acute Care Forum

CONTEXT

Acute Care Forums (ACFs) are one of the key ways in which the recommendations in the policy implementation guide and other service improvements are actioned and delivered. The membership of ACFs ideally includes a broad range of representative people such as service users and carers, ward staff, senior professional leads, community acute care representatives and others. The National Institute for Mental Health in England has downloadable information on The Capable Acute Care Forum (http://www.londondevelopmentcentre.org/resource/local/docs/CAPABLE_ ACUTE_CARE_FORUM.doc).

In our survey we wanted to find out whether Acute Care Forums had been developed in all trusts and whether ward managers felt that they could influence them.

WHAT WE FOUND

In total, 94% (298 responses) of ward managers confirmed that there was an Acute Care Forum (ACF) in their trust. In the East Midlands and Eastern regions this figure was 100%. The remaining regions all had some trusts where ward managers reported that ACFs were not in operation. Nonetheless these findings are very encouraging and show how much development has occurred since 2002 when ACFs were recommended in the *Mental Health Policy Implementation Guide: Adult Acute Inpatient Care Provision* (DH, 2002a).

As well as just knowing numbers, we wanted to find out whether ward managers felt that they could influence the ACF and we found that 88% of ward managers felt that they could. However, across all regions 32 ward managers stated that they felt they could not influence their ACF. In the Eastern region, 33% (7 ward managers) stated that they could not influence the ACF and, as a percentage of those that took part in the survey, this was higher than all other regions.

Figure 85   If you have an Acute Care Forum can you influence it? (273 responses)

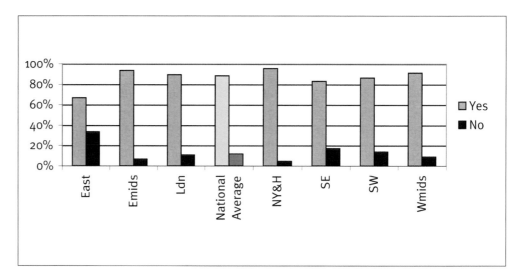

RECOMMENDATIONS

Reviews ❖ RDCs and ACFs should work together in reviewing the findings in this report.

❖ RDCs, particularly Eastern region, should work with ACFs to explore and understand what prevents ward managers from influencing the ACF and to develop strategies to improve communications.

Implementation ❖ ACFs should devise action plans to assist and facilitate the implementation of recommendations in the MH-PIG Adult Acute.

❖ ACFs should develop strategies to ensure the delivery of service improvement plans.

Monitoring ❖ RDCs should work with ACFs to monitor the implementation of the guidance recommendations.

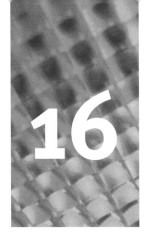

16 Concluding remarks

The *Acute Care 2004* national benchmarking survey consisted of two postal questionnaires: one sent to every ward manager in England and the other to every NHS trust providing acute mental health inpatient care. While not every ward manager or trust responded, most did, and thanks to this we have a substantive picture of acute inpatient provision across England. Obviously the confidence we can have in the findings is moderated by the response rate and this varies considerably by region.

The *Acute Care 2004* survey in large part presents the perspectives and experience of inpatient care and provision of those working in these services; and we do not claim that the survey is in any way a definitive picture. Any project must set itself limits and the limits we set meant that the views and experiences of those who use inpatient services and those who work in partnership with them have not been surveyed as part of this project (though service users' comments have been sought throughout the project). When comparing the managers' perceptions gathered in our survey with the service users' perceptions in the recent Mind *Ward Watch* report (Mind, 2004), our own service user feedback and other reports, it is notable that there are some very important differences particularly around safety and environment. These discrepancies tell us much about where the gaps are and give a clear indication of action needed to close them. We suggest that further research should include the views of service users to ensure that a more complete picture is achieved.

These limitations notwithstanding, the survey has produced a useful and indeed large body of findings. The intention of the survey was to produce 'benchmarks' with which services could compare themselves. Although some 'benchmarks' proved elusive, the survey has been successful in generating a considerable number. Just three examples are: indicators of 'continuity of care' such as average weekly agency nursing hours; indicators of quality of care such as the access to leisure activities and therapies; and indicators of user engagement such as the checklist of available information for service users and the checklist of user involvement methods.

Additionally, at the national and regional levels, the various 2002/2003 Hospital Episode Statistics we have presented provide a benchmark of acute care before the *National Service Framework for Mental Health* (DH, 1999a) was implemented in earnest. This will be invaluable to help to measure the success of that implementation in the coming years.

A survey of this sort raises as many questions as it set out to answer and these too are useful in that they suggest specific areas for further work. Some ward managers (a significant minority) have reported their perception that the implementation of crisis resolution teams (CRTs) has had an impact on the profile of service users being admitted, in that they have noticed an increase in their severity of mental health problems. This is perhaps a predictable result of successful CRT implementation (keeping all but the most acutely unwell out of hospital) and should be tested more rigorously. Such a change may provide a useful indicator of successful CRT implementation, but also requires those providing services to consider how they might prepare ward staff for dealing with a greater severity of illness amongst service users.

The inpatient ward is part of a system of care and its links with other parts of that system are crucial to the well being of the people served by that system. The commentary on communication between community teams and inpatient services is particularly useful here. The findings suggest that there is considerable room for improvement and further surveying is necessary to look more deeply at this issue. Given its importance, some 'harder' indicators (we have measured ward managers' perceptions and reported experience) could be developed here.

The report has been divided into themed chapters for ease of use and each chapter has key findings and recommendations which we developed in collaboration with people working in acute care and other acknowledged experts in the field. We believe these provide a useful tool in that they provide prompts and questions that should support the monitoring of these services and promote improvement. However, to make best use of these findings and recommendations we would urge that they are considered and explored in the context of the rest of the system of mental health care, not in isolation. We would also advise the involvement of service users in exploring and looking at ways to address the issues raised.

The *Acute Care 2004* survey is the first exercise of its kind and has occurred at quite a critical time in the implementation of the various reforms that emerged from the NSF-MH. It is intended as a starting point and this brief commentary has given just a few examples of how it can be taken further.

Acute inpatient care remains a vital part of any mental health system. Yet it is too often neglected in favour of the growing ranks of community services. This survey indicates how much still needs to be achieved in improving acute care services to meet the ambitions we all have for the service we want to see.

Appendix 1

International Statistical Classification of Diseases and Related Health Problems
– 10th Revision, Version for 2003

Taken from the World Health Organisation website
http://www.who.int/classifications/icd/en/

Tabular List of inclusions and four-character subcategories

Chapter V: Mental and behavioural disorders
(F00-F99)

F00-F09	Organic, including symptomatic, mental disorders
F10-F19	Mental and behavioural disorders due to psychoactive substance use
F20-F29	Schizophrenia, schizotypal and delusional disorders
F30-F39	Mood [affective] disorders
F40-F48	Neurotic, stress-related and somatoform disorders
F50-F59	Behavioural syndromes associated with physiological disturbances and physical factors
F60-F69	Disorders of adult personality and behaviour
F70-F79	Mental retardation
F80-F89	Disorders of psychological development
F90-F98	Behavioural and emotional disorders with onset usually occurring in childhood and adolescence
F99	Unspecified mental disorder

Appendix 2

Organisation of HES data by International Classification of Diseases, 10th revision
(ICD10) codes into psychosis and non-psychosis

ICD10 CODE	DIAGNOSIS
Psychosis related	
F20 – F20.9, F25 – F25.9	Schizophrenic Disorders
F30 – F31.9	Affective Psychoses
F10.5, F12.5, F13.5, F14.5, F15.5, F16.5, F17.5, F18.5, F19.5, F21.X – F24.X, F28.X – F29.X, F32.3, F33,3, F34.1	Other Psychoses (Including drug & alcohol induced)
Non-psychosis related	
F00.0 – F03.X	Dementia
F04.X – F09.X, F62 – F99.X	Other Diagnoses
F10 – F10.4, F10.6 – F12.4, F12.6 – F13.4, F13.6 – F14.4, F14.6 – F15.4, F15.6 – F16.4, F16.6 – F17.4, F17.6 – F18.4, F18.6 – F19.4, F19.6 – F19.9	Drug/Alcohol Disorders
F32 – F32.2, F32.8 – F33.2, F33.4 – F33.9, F40 – F41.9	Anxiety/Depression
F34 – F34.0, F34.8 – F39.X, F42 – F59.X	Other Neurotic
F60 – F61.X	Personality Disorders

Appendix 3

Percentage of Finished Consultant Episodes by ethnic group								
	East %	E Mids %	London %	NW %	NY&H %	SE %	S %	W Mids %
White:								
British	67.16	65.80	54.25	68.92	70.04	60.24	68.72	67.02
Irish	0.55	0.70	1.16	0.67	0.64	0.61	0.59	0.76
Any other white background	6.29	3.05	8.61	3.58	5.12	5.36	3.40	3.61
Mixed:								
White and Black Caribbean	0.25	0.19	0.44	0.18	0.26	0.19	0.22	0.25
White and Black African	0.07	0.06	0.21	0.08	0.10	0.12	0.13	0.12
White and Asian	0.10	0.08	0.22	0.11	0.13	0.12	0.14	0.15
Any other mixed background	0.12	0.14	0.26	0.12	0.15	0.14	0.14	0.15
Asian or Asian British:								
Indian	1.23	1.28	2.70	1.06	1.44	1.07	1.28	1.29
Pakistani	0.67	0.72	1.23	0.72	0.83	0.87	0.64	0.77
Bangladeshi	0.32	0.23	0.68	0.22	0.26	0.20	0.22	0.37
Any other Asian background	0.37	0.36	0.80	0.35	0.26	0.29	0.28	0.44
Black or Black British:								
Caribbean	1.83	2.15	4.68	1.53	1.91	1.60	1.61	2.52
African	0.95	1.21	2.68	0.95	0.95	1.05	0.90	1.26
Any other Black background	0.86	1.05	1.83	0.79	0.89	0.94	0.65	0.96
Other Ethnic Groups:								
Chinese	0.17	0.15	0.42	0.17	0.16	0.17	0.20	0.20
Any other ethnic group	0.90	1.08	2.19	0.89	0.94	1.00	0.85	1.14
Not stated	18.16	21.77	17.65	19.67	15.92	26.02	20.04	18.99

Percentages calculated from Hospital Episode Statistics (DH, 2002-3) using categories as per the Data Set Change Notice 21/2000 (DH, 2000)

References

Bowers, L. (2003) Runaway patients. *Mental Health Practice,* **7** (1) 10–12.

Campbell, P. (2004) *How to cope with hospital admission.* London: Mind. (Available from www.mind.org.uk)

Care Programme Approach Association (2004) *The CPA Handbook.* Chesterfield: CPA Association.

Chahal, K. & Ullah, A.I. (2004) *Experiencing Ethnicity: Discrimination and Service Provision. Foundations report.* York: Joseph Rowntree Foundation.

Clarke, S. (2004) *Acute Inpatient Mental Health Care: Education, Training & Continuing Professional Development for All.* Leeds: NIMHE.

Department of Health (1999a) *National Service Framework for Mental Health: Modern Standards and Service Models for Mental Health.* London: DH. (Available from www.dh.gov.uk)

Department of Health (1999b) *Drug Misuse and Dependence: Guidelines on Clinical Management.* London: DH. (Available from www.dh.gov.uk)

Department of Health (1999c) *Effective care co-ordination in mental health services: modernising the care programme approach – a policy booklet.* London: DH. (Available from www.dh.gov.uk)

Department of Health (2000a) *The NHS Plan: a plan for investment, a plan for reform.* London: DH. (Available from www.dh.gov.uk)

Department of Health (2001a) *Mental health policy implementation guide.* London: DH. (Available from www.dh.gov.uk)

Department of Health (2001b) *Working together, learning together: a framework for lifelong learning for the NHS.* London: DH. (Available from www.dh.gov.uk)

Department of Health (2002a) *Mental health policy implementation guide: Adult Acute Inpatient Care Provision.* London: DH. (Available from www.dh.gov.uk)

Department of Health (2002b) *Mental health policy implementation guide: Dual diagnosis good practice guide.* London: DH. (Available from www.dh.gov.uk)

Department of Health (2002c) *Delivering 21st century IT support for the NHS: national strategic programme.* London: DH. (Available from www.dh.gov.uk)

Department of Health (2002d) *Mental health policy implementation guide: National minimum standards for general adult services in Psychiatric Intensive Care Units (PICU) and Low Secure Environments.* London: DH. (Available from from www.dh.gov.uk)

Department of Health (2003a) *Inside Outside: Improving Mental Health Services for Black and Minority Ethnic Communities in England.* London: DH (Available from www.dh.gov.uk)

Department of Health (2003b) *Mainstreaming gender and women's mental health: implementation guidance.* London: DH (Available from www.dh.gov.uk)

Department of Health (2003c) *Mental health services workforce design and development best practice guidance.* London: DH (Available from www.dh.gov.uk)

Department of Health (2004) *National Service Framework for Children, Young People and Maternity Services.* London: DH. (Available from www.dh.gov.uk)

Department of Health (2005) *Delivering Race Equality in Mental Health Care: An action plan for reform inside and outside services and the Government's response to the Independent inquiry into the death of David Bennett.* London: DH. (Available from www.dh.gov.uk)

Department of Health and Disability Rights Commission (2004) *Department of Health/Disability Rights Commission framework for partnership action on disability 2004/5.* London: DH. (Available from www.dh.gov.uk)

Ford, R., Durcan, G., Warner, L., Hardy, P., & Muijen, M. (1998) One day survey by the Mental Health Act Commission of acute adult psychiatric inpatient wards in England and Wales. *British Medical Journal,* **317:** 1279–1283. (Available from http://bmj.bmjjournals.com)

Genkeer, L., Gough, P. & Finlayson, B. (2003) *London's Mental Health Workforce: A review of recent developments.* London: King's Fund. (Available from www.kingsfund.org.uk)

Glasby, J., & Lester, H. (2003) *Cases for Change 1–5: An overview of the evidence which is driving the agenda for change: Booklets 1–5.* Leeds: NIMHE. (Available from www.nimhe.org.uk)

Health and Social Care Advisory Service (HAS) (2003) *Improving the Quality of Psychiatric Inpatient Care in London (IQPIL).* Available from www.healthadvisoryservice.org/pdf_files/IQPIL%2oreport.pdf [Accessed 10 February 2005]

Healthcare Commission (2003) *What CHI has found in: mental health trusts. Sector report.* Available from: http://www.chi.nhs.uk/eng/cgr/mental_health/mental_health_report03.pdf [Accessed 10 February 2005]

Higgins, R., Hurst, K. & Wistow, G. (1999) *Psychiatric Nursing Revisited: The Mental Health Nursing Care Provided for Acute Psychiatric Patients.* London: Whurr Books.

Hoadley, A., Philip, M. & Dhillon, K. (2005, unpublished) *Scoping the current problems and solutions relating to consultant psychiatrist vacancies, consultant recruitment and the use of locums in England.* (Available from www.scmh.org.uk)

House of Commons Hansard Written Answer, 6 May 2004: Column 1811W. Available from: http://www.publications.parliament.uk/pa/cm200304/cmhansrd/vo040506/text/40506w46.htm#40506w46.html_sbhdo [Accessed 10 February 2005]

House of Commons Hansard Written Answer, 21 June 2004: Column 1275W. Available from: http://www.publications.parliament.uk/pa/cm200304/cmhansrd/vo040621/text/40621w29.htm#40621w29.html_sbhd1[Accessed 10 February 2005]

Kennedy, P., Lane, E., Williams, C., Brown, M., Niemic, S., Tacchi, M-J. & Smyth, M. (2003) *More than the sum of all the parts: Improving the whole system with Crisis Resolution and Home Treatment.* Available from: http://nimheneyh.org.uk/item.cfm?secid=27&subid=105&itemid=74 [Accessed 10 February 2005]

mentality (2003) *Not All in the Mind: The physical health of mental health service users. Briefing paper 2.* London: mentality.

Mind (2004) *Ward Watch: Mind's campaign to improve hospital conditions for mental health patients.* London: Mind

Morris, J. (2004) *One town for my body, another for my mind: Services for people with physical impairments and mental health support needs.* York: Joseph Rowntree Foundation. (Available from www.jrf.org.uk)

National Audit Office (2003) *A Safer Place to Work: Protecting NHS Hospital and Ambulance Staff from Violence and Aggression.* Report by the Comptroller and Auditor General HC 527 Session 2002-2003: 27 March 2003. London: NAO. (Available from www.nao.org.uk)

National Institute for Clinical Excellence (2005) *Violence: The short-term management of disturbed/violent behaviour in in-patient psychiatric settings and emergency departments. Clinical Guidelines 25.* London: NICE. (Available from www.nice.org.uk)

National Institute for Mental Health in England (2003a) *Engaging and Changing: Developing effective policy for the care and treatment of Black and minority ethnic detained patients.* Leeds: NIMHE. (Available from www.nimhe.org.uk)

National Institute for Mental Health in England (2003b) *Real Voices: Survey Findings from a series of community consultation events involving Black and minority ethnic groups in England.* Leeds: NIMHE. (Available from www.nimhe.org.uk)

National Institute for Mental Health in England (2004) *Mental health policy implementation guide: Developing positive practice to support the safe and therapeutic management of aggression and violence in mental health in-patient settings.* Leeds: NIMHE. (Available from www.nimhe.org.uk)

National Treatment Agency for Substance Misuse (2002) *Models of care for treatment of adult drug misusers. Part 1: Summary for commissioners and managers responsible for implementation.* London: NTA. (Available from www.nta.nhs.uk)

National Treatment Agency for Substance Misuse (2002) *Models of care for the treatment of drug misusers. Part 2: Full reference report.* London: NTA (Available from www.nta.nhs.uk)

NHS Executive (2000) *Safety, privacy and dignity in mental health units: guidance on mixed sex accommodation for mental health services.* London: DH. (Available from www.dh.gov.uk)

Northern Centre for Mental Health (2003) *National Continuous Quality Improvement Tool for Mental Health Education.* Available from the NIMHE North East, Yorkshire & Humber Development Centre: http://nimheneyh.org.uk/subject.cfm?secid=27&subid=108 [Accessed 10 February 2005]

Quirk, A. & Lelliott, P. (2001) What do we know about life on acute psychiatric wards in the UK? A review of the research evidence. *Social Science & Medicine,* **53**, 1565-1574.

Quirk, A. & Lelliot, P. (2004) Users' experiences of in-patient services. In: Campling, P., Davies, S., & Farquharson, G. (eds) *From Toxic Institutions to Therapeutic Environments: Residential Settings in Mental Health Services.* London: Gaskell Publications.

Rose, D. (2001) *Users' Voices: The perspectives of mental health service users on community and hospital care.* London: SCMH

Royal College of Psychiatrists (1998a) *Not Just Bricks and Mortar: Report of the Royal College of Psychiatrists Working Party on the size, staffing, structure, siting and security of new acute adult psychiatric inpatient units.* London: Royal College of Psychiatrists. (Available from www.rcpsych.ac.uk)

Royal College of Psychiatrists (1998b) *Psychiatric Beds and Resources: Factors Influencing Bed Use and Service Planning.* London: Gaskell Publications.

Royal College of Psychiatrists (2003 and ongoing) *The National Audit of Violence: towards safer and more therapeutic residential care for people with mental health problems or learning disability.* Unpublished.

Royal College of Psychiatrists (2004) *The National Audit of Violence, Newsletter Edition 6.* Unpublished.

Ryan, T. (2003) *A Survey of NW Acute Ward Managers: Supporting Acute Care Forums' service development agenda.* Feedback paper. Available from: tony@ryan1999.fsnet.co.uk

Sathyamoorthy, G., Minghella, E., Robertson, D., Bhui, K., & Ford, R. (2001) *Cultural Sensitivity Audit Tool for Mental Health Services.* London: SCMH.

The Sainsbury Centre for Mental Health (1998) *Acute Problems: A survey of the quality of care in acute psychiatric wards.* London: SCMH.

The Sainsbury Centre for Mental Health (2002) *Breaking the Circles of Fear: A review of the relationship between mental health services and African and Caribbean communities.* London: SCMH.

University of Durham (ongoing) *Adult Mental Health Service Mapping.* Available from: www.dur.ac.uk/service.mapping/amh [Accessed 10 February 2005]

Worrall, A., O'Herlihy, A., Banerjee, S., Jaffa, T., Lelliott, P., Hill, P., Scott, A. & Brook, H. (2004) Inappropriate admission of young people with mental disorder to adult psychiatric wards and paediatric wards: cross sectional study of six months' activity. *British Medical Journal,* **328**, 867. (Available from http://bmj.bmjjournals. com)